Addiction:
A Family Affair

The University of Florida
Guide to Understanding, Prevention,
and Dealing with Addiction

Scott A. Teitelbaum, M.D.
F.A.A.P., F.A.S.A.M.

Addiction:
A Family Affair

The University of Florida
Guide to Understanding, Prevention,
and Dealing with Addiction

ISBN-13: 9780983688204

Library of Congress-in-Publication Data

Cover and book design by PanoGraphics
Printed and bound in the USA by Selby Marketing
Editorial Services: Lawrence D. Chilnick

The information in this book is only for educational purposes. It is not
intended to replace the advice of a physician or medical practitioner. Consult
with a qualified healthcare provider before beginning any new health program,
medication or supplement.

McKnight Brain Institute
Department of Psychiatry
100 S Newell Drive L4-100
PO Box 100256
Gainesville, Fl 32610-0256

http://drscottteitelbaum.com/
www.FRC@psychiatry.ufl.edu

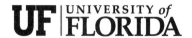

Dedication

To Daniel and Diane, my loving parents who provided and continue to provide inspiration in my life.

To my children, Sarah, Eric, Jacob, and Dahlia who are my greatest blessings. Words cannot describe my love for them.

To my wife and best friend Kim, who is the angel in my life.

To my brother and sister, Larry and Judi, who I dearly love.

Finally, to all the people, both addicts and family who have been touched by the disease of addiction but struggle every day to overcome their illness.

Acknowledgements

Writing this book was a group effort that required support and input and insight from many people. All stepped up to help me and were always willing to help. Larry Chilnick and Paula Edge's superb editorial skills helped me shape this book significantly.

Connie Pruitt, Marika Brigham, Tina Green and Priscilla Spence were there for me when I needed something for the book "yesterday". A special thanks to the talented artistic direction and design work to Rob Kalnitz and also to Rich Selby who has driven this project to help us make the deadline.

Also invaluable were the skill and talents of the FRC staff, because success in addiction treatment is also a team effort not an individual event.

Contents

Section I:
Your Family and Addiction

Section II:
A Guide to the Most Abused, Dangerous or Beneficial Drugs

Section III:
The UF Prevention and Treatment Methods

Foreword

Tobacco, alcohol, drugs of abuse, and misuse of prescription medications are the nation's number one health problem. These "diseases" often begin in adolescence and are the hardest to treat. They are also the most commonly ignored by health professionals, parents, and policy makers, buried in denial and lack of accurate information.

The tar and other chemicals in cigarettes increases a smoker's risk of lung cancer, emphysema, and bronchial disorders significantly; yet, rather than think about cigarettes and cigarette smoking, we developed very sophisticated treatments for lung cancer, emphysema, and bronchitis.

Binge drinking has become common on college campuses and among young adults. Rather than develop effective strategies for dealing with alcohol and alcohol-related problems, we have developed a "schizoid" system with law enforcement and DUIs on the one hand and liver transplants on the other.

We do not even check blood or breath alcohol on all emergency admissions for fear that we will have to take so many keys and keep so many under observation that we will strain an already broken emergency system.

For illicit drugs like marijuana or cocaine, we have done even worse. We have drug testing, drug courts, and jail. We do not have much in the way of "hands-on" addiction training for our health professionals, medical students, residents, nurses, and others; however, we actually train all physicians to deliver a baby, in spite of the fact that few, if any physicians ever deliver a baby again after medical school and only 2% of the medical school class will go into OB. No one seems to want to ask about drugs for fear they will not know what to do next.

All physicians will see alcohol abusers-addicts, drug abusers-addicts, medication mis-users-addicts in their practice, clinic or hospital. Yet virtually none of these are prepared to deal with a patient who clearly has addictive behavior. Only one medical school, UF (University of Florida), has a mandatory medical school clerkship experience, so that all students will get textbook and real-life practical competencies in addiction detection, management, and recovery.

With such poor training, it is no wonder that only 5% of all patients in treatment for addiction in Philadelphia, Pennsylvania were referred by an emergency room or physician.

Physicians usually pride themselves in making a diagnosis, giving advice, making an intervention and matching the patient with the appropriate treatment or specialist.

In a well developed, multi-level addiction medicine program:

- The family is the physician
- The family makes the assessment
- The family makes the intervention and
- The family sends the patient for an evaluation or on to treatment

While we fix medical education, the burden falls on the mothers and fathers to prevent abuse, dependence, and their consequences.

Tobacco, alcohol, or drug problems do not just happen one day. They start in the teenage years, when the brain is still developing and ripening. Smoke as a teen and you're likely to be a life-long smoker and addict. Binge drink as a teen and you are much more likely to have alcohol problems as an adult. Misuse prescription medications and you are more likely to have drug problems as a teen and thereafter.

This book is an in-depth family manual and resource. It provides empowering information from the world-class expert, pediatrician and addiction specialist, Scott Teitelbaum, MD. I could not think of a better person and addiction treatment expert to write such a family guide!

Dr. Teitelbaum has evaluated thousands of patients and families from around the USA, including physicians, who had the disease of addiction. He has treated the high and mighty and also the 'mighty high' with compassion, respect, and untiring energy. Nevertheless, no matter how successful Florida Recovery Center (FRC) or the Betty Ford Center is in evaluation, treatment and recovery, prevention is the only 100% effective treatment. Family education, dinners, family honesty, and family resistance training are the answer …not serving drinks to minors at home.

This book offers help and hope to families in dealing with the nation's, our nation's , number one health problem. Dr. Teitelbaum helps shine a bright light on this subject and busts myths and denial along the way. Treatment works, but prevention and when that fails early interventions, works the best... I may be biased, but n*o home should be without this book.* Read this book and pass it around to your family.

> *Mark S. Gold, M.D.*
> Distinguished Professor
> Donald R. Dizney Eminent Scholar
> University of Florida College of Medicine and
> McKnight Brain Institute
> Departments of Psychiatry, Neuroscience,
> Anesthesiology, Community Health & Family Medicine
> Chairman, Department of Psychiatry

Introduction:

How To Use This Book To Save Your Family

Have you ever asked yourself where all those pill bottles in the medicine cabinet came from? What are these pills for and should you keep them around for future use—save a little money if your toothache returns? What about that cough medicine—still some left in the bottle in case your cold returns? And that red pill, can you take it with a glass of wine? Or, are you trying to figure out where you can get some more of those "muscle relaxants" that your doctor gave you when you hurt your back slipping on the ice?

You are not at all alone when you are confused or wary about prescription and other abused drugs because literally, almost everyone is taking them. We use more every day as we get older (and in increasing numbers) with new drugs appearing on the market frequently. If you are part of a family of four or six, at least two or three of the adults or children in the family will take at least one prescription medication annually. It is likely you may also be faced with one of the puzzling situations above.

According to a variety of Federal agencies, including the Centers for Disease Control and Prevention (commonly referred to as the CDC), "Prescription drug use is rising among people of all ages, and use increases with age. Five out of six persons 65 and older are taking at least one medication and almost half the elderly take three or more."

The University of Florida Guide to Understanding, Prevention, and Dealing with Addiction is a manual that no home should be without for managing prescription, so-called recreational drugs, alcohol abuse and related mental health issues. Led by Scott Alan Teitelbaum, M.D., UF's Division of Addiction Medicine Chief and over 18 UF M.D's, who specialize in the entire spectrum of addiction treatment, every question and situation is either addressed in this book or can be found on our website or by contacting our clinic for an appointment with one of our specialists.

The UF Approach To Prevention, Treatment, and Recovery

The UF Guide explains one of the most important approaches to resolving drug and alcohol addiction, developed over the past four decades and clears myths that surround others:

- *Drug and alcohol addiction is a chronic disease in the same manner as a cardio-vascular event, type-2 diabetes, or hypertension. These diseases share similar characteristics with addiction, such as susceptibility caused by genetic history, clear pathophysiologic organ changes, and/or sociocultural problems. Further, a significant behavioral change is required to recover and return to health in each situation.*

- *There is no addiction "cure" like many other chronic diseases, but UF has developed multiple treatment methods and recovery strategies that blend the spiritual principles of Alcohol Anonymous, cognitive behavioral therapy, and modern psychopharmacology.*

The University of Florida and Florida Recovery Center program has been demonstrated to work in scientific studies published in the medical literature. In a recent study by NIDA founding Director Robert L. DuPont, M.D., over 80% recovery after treatment was found, even after a 5-year follow-up.

Essentially, the UF program challenges a patient in this way:

"Your brain may have been hijacked by a drug, but recovery must involve healing of the heart and soul."
Then it is your turn to work with the doctors, nurses, and therapists and overcome the odds.

This book is your standard reference to ensure the family's safe drug use through education and action. It is also a "database" for your family when a quick answer to a drug issue arises.

Section I: Your Family and Prescription Drugs

Each chapter in Section I will give you personal tools to cope with prescription drug misuse, abuse, and addiction.

What's Included:
- A report on surprising trends in dangerous drug abuse by different adolescent economic groups.
- What is addiction? Addiction 101 for anyone.
- How drug addiction has become more virulent among certain adult age groups.
- A history of drug addiction from ancient Egypt to the 21st Century to add context to the overall information in this book.
- How you and your family should approach medication.
- What are basic rules for the home?
- Talking to your M.D. about medication to avoid catastrophe.
- If it is in the drugstore, is it safe? Over-the counter-danger zones.
- Can parents increase family risk if they use medications frequently?
- Obvious safety steps but special measures to take (i.e. anaphylactic shock).

Section II:
A Guide To The Most Abused, Dangerous, Or Beneficial Drugs

This segment is not simply a typical compendium of medication profiles with endless "possible" side effects or directions and dosage information. Today virtually all prescriptions you have filled at the pharmacy come with patient information and most pharmacists can answer questions. Most important for you and your family is that this section of the *UF Guide* is focused extensively on medications that people are using with unrecognized (or purposely ignored) potential for addiction.

This segment of the *UF Guide* explains medications through "classes" of prescription medications that are dangerous, legal, and illegal and how this peril can be avoided. Each drug profile explains why certain prescription drugs can lead to dependence while others are safer. Medications and categories described in depth include:

- Alcohol
- Cocaine
- Marijuana
- Prescription Medications
- Over-The-Counter Products
- Inhalants
- Club Drugs/MDMA
- Heroin
- Hallucinogens
- Anabolic Steroids
- Tobacco
- Synthetic Marijuana
- Stimulants

Section III of this book describes UF prevention and multi-phase treatment methods told through actual case histories.

The overall goal of this book is to bring both the benefits of understanding and preventing addiction, the power of addiction and the drugs that can cause it. Add to that information that helps put it in the context of your life and your family will be safer.

The potential for problems with medications is the classic "good news/bad news" situation that we face as a nation that depends on prescription medications that have saved and extended the lives of millions. You cannot take it seriously enough. And, of course prescription drugs are a significant part of the economy mostly because they can be counted on to increase in sales every year. In fact while health care costs rose by almost 10% in the past several years, medication costs rose 15%-40% depending on the category of drug. The really bad news is that the level of prescription drug abuse is also growing considerably.

Each year, the Federal Government agency, Substance Abuse and Mental Health Services Administration (SAMHSA) conducts an extensive survey of drug use of all kinds of people, aged 12 and older. This study is known as the National Survey on Drug Use and Health (NSDUH). They reported that almost 7% of people (12 and up) had used mental health medications (i.e. Adderall—a combo stimulant for ADHD) in the prior month—for something other than what they were prescribed for such as pain killers, sedation or stimulation. Other statistics show the same sort of drug abuse over the past several years among adolescents.

You will also find in-depth information and statistics from this survey and also another well regarded study: Monitoring The Future (conducted by the University of Michigan Institute for Social Research at the request of NIDA) that has tracked adolescent drug abuse for decades. These give you an idea of how teens perceive the danger of drugs.

Is America the most medicated nation on Earth?—asks the CDC in its report. While most of the pills are beneficial—reducing cholesterol and heart disease—misuse is all too common as you'll see in the next chapter—**Drug Abuse Trends Today: What You Really Don't Know.** What's included?

- Why today's drug abuse trends are not like the '60's or even the '80's
- OTC's and Teens—Today's surprise about "addiction and substances of abuse" in different teens groups (plus other trends from UF, The U Michigan Study—Why there is a difference among adolescents groups)
- The issues surrounding M.D. and pharmacy shopping put the abuse of medication into an entirely new world.
- A history of drug use and addiction.
- The "new" definition of addiction
- Who uses the most drugs today

Chapter One:

Drug Abuse Trends Today: What You Really Don't Know

This book is a red flag waving at anyone who faces the challenges of raising a family in the 21st century, keeping everyone healthy and sober. The stress we face as adults can quickly lead to drug or alcohol dependency and this book serves as a roadmap to prevent that disaster. *The UF Guides* help you hold it all together.

Our children are under severe pressure to succeed and often they are on their own while parents may be absent working long hours. Truthfully, all of us lead vulnerable lives. It is hardly surprising that 23.6 million persons aged 12 or older needed treatment for an illicit drug or alcohol abuse problem in just a single year.

The US spends $40 billion each year on drug control despite the fact that there are multiple studies of far less expensive ways to attack drug use and educate our children.

In fact the total cost to our economy from drug abuse and addiction is growing far beyond the days when "stoner movies" and Studio 54 defined "recreational drugs." Cost to our country—alone—is estimated at $510.8 billion. The Rand Corporation estimates that an effective drug prevention program could be provided for 3.75 million seventh graders at $150 each—or only $550 million per year. Why aren't we doing this?

A second red flag is flying and signifies that many adults and baby boomers are actually clueless about today's "supercharged" version of well known abused drugs. The information in this chapter may shock some people who will learn that not only is the "drug problem" in the U.S. different now, but time really flew by and we never noticed it! We were growing up, but some remained behind or came in contact with substances for our tennis elbow and something that would help us bill out at maximum $$$ per hour. This book will explain it.

New drugs and patterns of drug abuse and addiction today bear little similarity to those of the boomers or GenXers, just now having families. For example, the same brand name hallucinogens (Purple Haze, LSD) that the Flower Children tripped on and danced to in the parks of San Francisco are only a memory. Pot is still very widely used, but now we have "medical marijuana" a carefully cultivated hybrid far more powerful than the "Woodstock generation dope" and dispensed in actual *Drug Stores* and farm markets. Heroin is no longer the drug of choice for only "beat poets" and jazz musicians favored in the coffee houses of Greenwich Village. Nor is the drinking on college campuses the same harmless "fun" as the Frat House beer busts and toga parties so perfectly filmed in the legendary *Animal House*. Blind drunk literally seems to be the goal, while downing a dozen "jello shots" has replaced such "high end" vintages like Mateus which we also used as candle holders.

Alcohol & Public Health Binge Drinking According to the CDC:

Binge drinking is a common pattern of excessive alcohol use in the United States. The National Institute on Alcohol Abuse and Alcoholism defines binge drinking as a pattern of drinking that brings a person's blood alcohol concentration (BAC) to 0.08 grams percent or above. This typically happens when men consume 5 or more drinks, and when women consume 4 or more drinks, in about 2 hours. Most people who binge drink are not alcohol dependent.

- Approximately 92% of U.S. adults who drink excessively report binge drinking in the past 30 days.
- College students commonly binge drink, but 70% of binge drinking episodes involve adults aged 26 years and older.
- The prevalence of binge drinking among men is higher than the prevalence among women.
- Binge drinkers are 14 times more likely to report alcohol-impaired driving than non-binge drinkers.
- About 90% of the alcohol consumed by youth under the age of 21 in the United States is in the form of binge drinks.

Despite publicity and indisputable scientific evidence that tie it to lung cancer, heart disease, diabetes, and hypertension, cigarette smoking keeps its users both physically and psychologically addicted. Most recent statistics indicate that 24.8 % of the male population smokes and 18.3 % of females smoke. There are literally thousands of stop smoking programs—but none really succeed.

"I can't stop, I tried," is the ultimate form of denial because the truth about cigarettes is that smoking is so effective as a "delivery system" that it is like an IV without the needle. Smoking is the fastest way to deliver a drug to the brain.

Today's cigarettes are not that different from previous generations' despite the marketing—but we know so much more today. You would think we'd gotten smarter! That's the real change in cigarette use—the addictive nature of nicotine is understood, but is without an effective method of stopping, except "cold turkey." Unfortunately, especially with cigarettes, relapse is one of the characteristics of recovery.

Treatment programs for nicotine also know that one real problem is that "smoking" has an image attached to it that either appeals to some people or not. Many smokers still associate activities with smoking like sitting in a bar or (yes) post sex that are so fixed in their minds that relearning to carry out some simple tasks is necessary.

Billions of $$ Can't Stop Teen Smoking!

Cigarette smoking, targeted for massive education programs and virtually banned everywhere, still continues among young people, especially females. The American Lung Association estimates that:

> *"Every minute four thousand eight hundred teens will take their first drag off a cigarette. Of those four thousand eight hundred, about two thousand will go on to be chain smokers. The fact that teen smoking rates are steadily increasing is disturbing. We are finding out that about 80% of adult smokers started smoking as teenagers." (see Section III)*

Drug use for Boomers back in the '60's and '70's --was often a college activity with two memorable mantras for the ultimate lifestyle: "sex, drugs & rock'n roll", or "turn on, tune in, & drop out" for those who preferred hallucinogens.

The drug picture at our universities today does not center on a way of life, or a central binding cause like an unpopular war. Higher education is serious—the US has the highest percentage of its population attending college. Keeping them healthy and sober is critical.

Even the elderly, who now live longer, are abusing prescription and over the counter drugs. According the National Institute on Drug Abuse (NIDA), persons 65 years of age and above comprise only 13 percent of the population, yet they account for approximately one-third of all medications prescribed in the United States. Older patients are more likely to be prescribed long-term and multiple prescriptions, which can lead to unintentional misuse. The elderly also are at risk for prescription drug abuse, in which they intentionally take medications that are not medically necessary.

If you think all of the above is from some sort of bizarre alternative universe, there are many more drugs that are either new or spin offs from medications that had been legal, but have become closely controlled substances and sources of serious health consequences, crime, and violence. For example:

- Amphetamines (Adderall, dexedrine, Ritalin)

- Methamphetamines (home brewed)

- Club drugs (MDMA, roofies, ecstacy)

- Ketamine (animal tranquilizers)

- PCP (angel dust)

- Over The Counter drugs (triple c's, dextromethorphan)

- Mescaline (psilocybin, magic mushrooms)

- Anabolic steroids

- Human growth hormones

- Prescription pain relievers and antidepressants (oxycodone, benzodiazepines, barbiturates)

The list goes on, although compared to the damage caused by the 50,000 naturally occurring toxins in our environments, the abused and addictive drugs are a far smaller group. Toxic pollution is a very serious public health problem, but the major catch is that drugs leading to addiction can do so quickly and the neurological damage is frequently permanent.

 On the other hand, if you live near a glowing swamp, or sparking electric cables, you can always move.

Today, drug abuse is so widespread that entering a rehab as a professional, M.D., executive, elected official, or high-visibility athlete or entertainer seems to be a seal of approval by tolerant audiences who see them as role models for beating drugs. This is not totally outside the box. It is almost like there is a celeb of the month club in rehab. But they are simply one more individual facing the nature of a death threat from the 21st century circumstances of drug abuse. UF has responded in a manner that is effective and discussed in more depth in **Section III.**

Despite the new challenge for addiction specialists at UF, their philosophy is that the person using the drug is not the problem—the drug is. This sounds like giving the user a free pass, but it is not.

*First, the power of today's drugs is a legitimate roadblock. Which of your receptor sites does a drug you've started to use turn on? Second, treatment can be impacted by many things; for example, your family situation (history of alcoholism or physical abuse). We also want to know how and why the drug that has you hooked is riding your brain's pathways to your most vulnerable receptor sites. The method to treat drug addiction in the new millennium is **NOT** to blame the addict, but free him or her from the drugs' psychological and neurological power.*

There are several key reasons that drug abuse in the 21st Century is so virulent beyond the difference in the power of common drugs and pills for abuse, which are discussed in detail in **Section II.**

- Availability and the inability of the U.S. government and many others to prevent highly organized, violent, and global sources from penetrating our borders. Billions are spent in Mexico, South America and Asia, resulting only in more "collateral damage" to citizens and those in our military uniforms.

- A great deal of time and money has been spent studying drug abuse among high school students, college students, and 20-somethings. We have learned that if you and others begin using drugs at an earlier age, you are more likely to continue and as you reach high school, college and beyond, your peer group will also continue to use at the same rate.

- Students who use drugs frequently (about 15%) drop out and are not counted as part of the problem—or sadly a clear example of the damage of today's drugs.
- Unless you are involved in juvenile and family law, it is not likely that you will realize there are actually four "classes" of adolescent drug users: urban poor, street gangs, middle class, and insured addicts who can afford treatment.
- New products are being imported to expanding markets. There is probably a saturation point for your traditional "drugs of mass destruction" but the market has embraced narcotic prescription medication and created a gigantic demand. Add to that some home-made recipes of "speed" in the form of dangerous versions of crystal meth. Even moonshine is back.

- The most surprising is the stash you can get in your local pharmacy. Young and enterprising high school hustlers "make the rounds" and super store pharmacies get disco.

Chapter Two:

Addiction 101

This *Family Guide* focuses on helping you recognize the reality of the dangers of prescription drugs, other substances, and why. In fact, if you are reading this book you may already be concerned about a family member, child or friend. Your "gut" may be right. Unfortunately, UF's clinical experience and dozens of reports and studies show that drug abuse is similar in scope to the current epidemic level diseases of cardiovascular failure and diabetes. Ironically while more and more people are actually benefiting from new prescription medication, abuse of some old-school standards like the **opiate pain killers, alcohol, and marijuana** are still widely abused or rising, especially among teenagers.

Today, more **prescription pills** are frequently linked to addiction for both legally prescribed and illegally used medication for pain, stimulation, increased concentration, anxiety or depression. Anyone who is using prescription drugs, but then finds himself or herself drawn to them *after* they have completed treatment, may begin to use those pills in ways that eventually harms them. This is a serious red flag warning you of your potential for problems with future drug use.

The good news is that you can be treated successfully for abuse of medication, and so-called recreational drugs, through a variety of multi-phase approaches developed at UF that are targeted at the source of addiction. This program is fully explained beginning in **Section III.**

What Do We Mean Addicted?

Addiction has many definitions, from the "official" to the anecdotal results of certain negative and self-destructive behavior.

The American Society of Addiction Medicine (ASAM) — **the medical definition of the addiction physician's professional organization says:**

"*Addiction is a primary, chronic disease of brain reward, motivation, memory and related circuitry. Dysfunction in these circuits leads to characteristic biological, psychological, social and spiritual manifestations.*

This is reflected in an individual pathologically pursuing reward and/or relief by substance use and other behaviors.

"Addiction is characterized by inability to consistently abstain, impairment in behavioral control, and craving, diminished recognition of significant problems with one's behaviors and interpersonal relationships, and a dysfunctional emotional response. Like other chronic diseases, addiction often involves cycles of relapse and remission. Without treatment or engagement in recovery activities, addiction is progressive and can result in disability or premature death."

The American Psychiatric Association (APA) publishes the "official" classification criteria for mental health problems known as the *Diagnostic and Statistical Manual of Mental Disorders (DSM).* The DSM is revised and updated every few years. You can see the evolving definition of addiction as each new revision is released. The DSM system is also flexible, relying on a list of behaviors, but the patient has to only demonstrate that he or she is clearly involved in a portion of the criteria. The DSM's recent proposed changes are designed to make a diagnosis clearer, too. Among the changes, for example, the diagnosis of substance dependence (depending on a number of criteria) will be substance use disorder mild, moderate or severe. As of this time, DSM-V has not been released.

Other DSM addiction standards can be "a maladaptive pattern of substance-use leading to clinically significant impairment or distress, as manifested by two (or more)" of the criteria listed in the book. Most patients have to have a certain percentage of the standards. For that reason we consider a wide variety of criteria to develop a treatment program that makes an accurate diagnosis of addiction and subsequent care. Another might be "a pathological attachment marked by preoccupation with drugs and narrowing of interest in anything BUT drugs."

The reality is that your level of addiction is defined in many contexts—your behavior, your DNA and how your brain chemistry reacts to what you are taking. Here are some more ways to look at addiction in general before going into more depth:

- Let's start with this one that most will recognize from TV, film and other media: A drug addict is someone who "needs to score" drugs in lowest, dirty crack houses, and uses them in uncontrolled ways that might kill themselves, send them to sell their bodies on the street, or land them with a jail sentence. This is a partial truth that many people embrace to rationalize their own drug abuse claiming "I can stop anytime; I'm a user, not an abuser." These are proverbial final words, before going off the cliff into the abyss.

- Drug abuse, misuse, and "recreational" use are not as much about the demographics of the "user" but rather, about the effects of specific drugs and people's reaction to the drugs used. You can be a street person, blue collar worker, or Wall Street executive in today's drug filled environment. The exposure to a specific drug may set off a buzz or do nothing for you at all.

- Biological and neurological response and behavior towards different substances, not being a part of a stereotyped culture (i.e. poverty, race), can destroy a life through unintended over-use. For example, various people find themselves unable to stop misusing one substance (for example, pills that provide stimulation), but experience no problem stopping another (such as, tranquilizers or sedatives). Think of how people choose an ice cream cone—by taste and flavor.

- Another very common definition is a popular and simple one used by clinicians and applies to many people-- you are an addict if you continue to use a drug, alcohol, or medication despite the recognition (and fact) that it is harming you. Think of it this way-- abuse MAY lead to dependence that then equals abuse, leading to addiction. This is what occurs over time.

- While not a strict definition of addiction, the greater use of a "new legal" prescription drug in the population, can be a clear indicator that there are probably more people misusing these drugs than should be. Recent data released by the Centers for Disease Control (CDC) reinforces this trend.

"Among persons aged 12 or older who used pain relievers non-medically in the past 12 months, 56.5 percent reported that they got the drug from someone they knew and that they did not pay for it. a smaller group purchased the drugs from '*dealers*' and on the internet, but most got the drugs from others who legally obtained the drugs from a physician."

Another significant statistic that represents a marked change in adolescent drug addiction is that marijuana may not longer be the "gateway drug" for this group. Beginning in 2005, more teenagers began their drug use through an opioid drug like oxycodone.

Addiction: How It Works

There are two significant aspects of substance abuse disorders that are keys to understanding why most experts brand it a "disease." It is also true that some other experts do lay the blame at the feet of the user, family, genetics, sexual abuse, poverty, or too much money, as if addiction is a character defect. Below is a more accurate snapshot of how a person with **addictive-related behavior** acts and the essential symptoms that can provide clues for anyone concerned about someone's drug use. A simple way to sum it up is this: Addiction can also be seen as "a progression of liking, to wanting to needing."

First, and above all, addiction is a **"brain disease,"** regardless of whether your problem stems from taking too many pills, smoking marijuana, or crack-cocaine. Before going into great depth on the disease model of addiction, think of drug abuse as something similar to banging your head against the wall. Eventually you may stop or knock yourself out, and then you are luckily revived. Unfortunately, your pathways in the brain are crushed, changed forever. You may walk and talk, but every time you pass the same wall you feel a need to smack your head into it again despite no pleasure or reward. *You are sick.*

Keep in mind, though, that you are as responsible for recovery as any heart, high blood pressure, or diabetes patient or there will be unabated bad outcomes. Addiction can also, like these diseases, stem from brain changes, genetic predisposition. As with out-of-control diabetics, who have to control blood sugar levels, the addict has to manage his or her recovery behavior.

It is also very important to understand that of the many ways addiction is diagnosed; it is rarely the same for everyone. The symptoms for many are like those below and for just as many others they may not be evident at all to the user or their loved ones, who may simply think the ten bottles of pills found in their underwear drawer, are from different drug stores or doctors.

- From a behavioral view point, you are likely to have begun abusing a drug in a social situation. As the cliché goes, no one says, "I want to be a pill popping, heroin shooting, drug addict when I grow up."

- Another characteristic of the road to addiction is when you discover that before you know it, obtaining the drug is what your life has become about and nothing is more important--- not your kids' soccer games, work, sex, clean clothes, or even food. In short—you and your life are out of control— you are preoccupied, losing interest in everything around you, and most important, you often relapse (which is so frequent and expected that it is also part of the criteria for addiction.)

- Even if you have a bottomless bowl full of pills or another drug, it will never be enough because one guarantee the drug makes is that you will need more and more just to feel the way you did the first time you tried it. This is one of the most insidious aspects of addiction—a.k.a. **tolerance.**

- Another clear sign of actual addiction is the presence of what is commonly called **withdrawal,** from a drug. In the movies it is "cold turkey" where the crack head or alcoholic is tossed in a room and he or she spends days suffering from the worst flu-like symptoms anyone can imagine. The good news is that there is medication to alleviate some of the withdrawal symptoms today.

- There is also some dispute among addiction specialists whether withdrawal must be present to diagnose a pattern of drug use as addiction. *This is a widely believed public misconception.* **Withdrawal symptoms do not have to be present.** *In some cases after years of drug abuse, the brain is so damaged that they may finally appear.*

- However, some drugs produce withdrawal pains that can be quite dangerous and possibly fatal. There is no dispute that withdrawal and tolerance are not necessarily evident because tolerance reflects the neuro-adaptation—hold your liquor— consequence of what you are using.

- An extremely important consideration to keep in mind is this: you do not have to have both tolerance and withdrawal symptoms while on the substance you are abusing. It is neither sufficient nor necessary. One will be a strong indicator of addiction.

- Alcohol, opiates, and sedatives are most likely to provoke clear withdrawal symptoms when stopped.

- A final key point: The *sequence* in which any of the above manifests itself usually varies. However, one significant cause and effect is virtually always evident in addiction;

> **compulsivity to the point that your drug seeking or use continues despite horrible adverse effects such as** auto accidents, DUI's, stealing, medical complications, divorce, and financial ruin.

Why Addiction Is A Disease:

From the many symptoms and definitions of addiction above, you still might be persuaded that drug use leading to severe circumstances is intentional. After all, people volunteer for dangerous life style choices all of the time. Since no one aspires to drug addiction, is becoming a drug addict voluntary?

While someone may begin using drugs as a way to "chill-out," or get a buzz, one thing is inevitable: eventually, your brain itself sustains dramatic changes—your "wires" get crossed--- which is why you can build tolerance and dependence. You can begin to determine whether or not you may have the beginning of a problem if you find yourself frequently in the "party hearty" mode for a considerable period of time. BUT, if others around you come to the conclusion that the $250 DUI fine (with suspension of your license) is a bad choice and you still continue in the party mode, you have a problem.

As Robert L. DuPont, M.D. former head of the National Institute On Drug Abuse (NIDA) says, "You have developed a "hungry brain." Dr. DuPont also refers to this problem as a "selfish brain." As the brain changes, you will likely develop the compulsive behavior that can become so severe that many addicts may experience craving for a drug if they just drive by the location where they acquired their drugs or any pharmacy, as these literally cause biological triggers in the brain.

The new definitions by the American Psychiatric Association of drug addiction and our own experience at UF make it clear that drug abuse/addiction is a "chronic and relapsing illness." In other words, your drug use is a disease that occurs on a "continuum of maladaptive patterns" of use. This is why you can't stop. Your brain is captured and if for a number of reasons discussed below you have poorly controlled "addictive behavior," you will either stop or your addiction will deepen.

One of the other unfortunate aspects of the addict/non-addict (but still an abuser) is that those who can stop their excessive use of drugs and alcohol tend to be very judgmental.

What Exactly is a Disease? First, here is a baseline definition for disease to bring context to excessive drug use. According to the American Heritage Dictionary:

> "Disease is a pathological condition of a part, organ, or system of an organism resulting from various causes, such as infection, genetic defect, or environmental stress, and characterized by an identifiable group of signs or symptoms." (http://www.answers.com/topic/disease)

Another significant reason why most specialists feel that drug addiction is a disease is that there are many studies of brain activity that demonstrate how the normal pleasure and reward system causes significant changes in the brain's chemistry when using drugs. We all have a series of biological pathways in our brains that help regulate the pleasure/reward system that kicks in when we eat, have sex, exercise, or participate in any number of activities. These chemicals are needed to motivate us and regulate neurotransmitters involved in other more common activities like retention, learning, and memory.

Chemicals regulate each of these neurotransmitters; the ones most frequently mentioned are dopamine and serotonin. While dopamine is the major one, there may be hundreds and we still only know about 10% of them. The neurotransmitters also respond differently to the different types of drugs someone is taking. For example, when you use cocaine, your dopamine-reward pathway (a.k.a. the mesolimbicdopaminergic pathway) leads to a feeling of reward by influencing the levels of dopamine released.

This is when the brain is actually "hijacked." The brain-jacking drug jumps into the normal dopamine pathways and carries the drug to its normal receptor sites in the mid-brain where the motivation to get more because of the pleasure you feel is reinforced by the opioid receptors. If you can't get enough, the brain reward system will help you seek more.

There is also another consequence of using drugs to the point where you experience severe damage. When your brain becomes "rewired" by drugs, we now know that it is likely to sustain some level of permanent damage. Many scientists had suspected this; everyone knew that the brain changed after many years of tracking the brain through neuro and brain imaging. What has been discovered now is that these brain changes last weeks to months. Through cognitive testing, it has been shown that the changed brain has problems/difficulties in making certain judgments, in memory, and in processing speed. DNA may also a contributing factor. These can last for a very long time—days, months, years and forever.

The danger is always there. If an opiate addict has elective surgery they may be re-exposed and this can cause relapse. This may last and impede cognitive skills. Through all of the research done about drug addiction and its effects on the brain, one can see how drug addiction is considered a brain disease that is both disabling and ultimately can take your life, literally and figuratively.

One final note: Common among alcohol or drug addicts is this: there is always a sense of denial—at least in the beginning of treatment. Many have one great delusion; that they are able to control their use (despite the presence of a high level of addiction) without treatment. Denial is one of the great hallmarks of addiction.

Chapter Three-

Medicine & Addiction:
From Ancient Egypt To The 21ˢᵗ Century

To understand the growing problem of addiction to medications today, especially among adolescents and young people, it helps to know why there are so many opportunities (i.e. different types of pills, medications, plants, "herbs" and powerful liquids) for abuse. Why are there so many medications—many that were never intended for abuse until someone decided to try an "experiment" and then share it with a friend?

The primary answer is really simple: In the beginning, thousands of years ago, there was plenty of opportunity for those whose powers to heal were strong and the law of supply and demand was in play. Progress in medical development stopped and started as progressive civilizations flourished and then suddenly disappeared from a disease they had no immunity to or by simple slaughter. As you will see, pain killing opiates like morphine, mood altering drugs like cocaine or marijuana, and even alcohol were the basis for medical treatment for centuries. Even when "medications" like these work for many people, their addictive dangers may not be revealed until they are regulated after decades of use and unfortunate results.

Today these drugs are either illegal or only used infrequently because they have been replaced by less "dangerous" controlled medications. Medication use also tends to run in cycles and even their side effects may become a solution to another problem. This happens far more frequently than one would guess.

Three classic cases are Viagra, thalidomide, and Minoxidil.

- After decades of research, thalidomide was approved as a sleeping pill for pregnant women. Instead of bringing sleep, it resulted in thousands of horribly malformed babies.

- Minoxidil was a blood pressure control medication that had an unexpected, but a welcome side effect—it created hair regrowth for many people going bald.

- Everyone knows the "little blue pill" Viagra, which, along with other brands, was originally studied to be a combination blood pressure and angina treatment. Like minoxidil, it had a vasodilating effect, allowing certain arteries to fill with blood. In this case the engorged veins included the ones that created erections.

These are classic examples of a medication filling a consumer need, but of these three, one was a disaster. The other two have not been on the market that long and they are often used daily. Will they become medications that, as described in Chapter One, you have to have more and more regardless of the negative effect and potential damage to yourself?

Addiction, as described in Chapter Two, occurs along a spectrum of behavior and/or predisposition for different people. Once you begin you may not stop with "recreation." There are multiple neurological pathways leading to this end result that can put you in rehab or the morgue. From the stories of the medications above, you can understand why there is often controversy and blame around the industry today that creates and markets most medication—the pharmaceutical industry. Also known as "Big Pharma," it has been attacked frequently, as if they were manufacturing weapons of mass destruction. This is not accurate. There are two sides to this story.

- The pharmaceutical companies, despite strong regulation, continue to grow for many fundamental reasons; a very high percentage of medications do not provoke any sort of psychological reaction yet treat disease successfully.

- While there can be new drugs that turn out to be less effective than promised or can demonstrate potential serious interactions with food or other drugs, when used correctly, most drugs are safe and go through many test levels before being allowed on the U.S. market.

- Our drug regulations are not more stringent than many other countries and in fact, what might bring only a light sentence in the USA can bring very harsh sentences in many countries, especially the Middle East. This goes for both pharmaceuticals you obtain without a prescription and recreational drugs. (**See Section II for more info.**)

The reality is that Big Pharma has had an enormous impact on world health for more than a century, increasing longevity and improving our quality of life. Some studies report that medication has not just controlled disease, but extended our lives by at least two years. In fact, the US economy currently has net gains of an estimated $2.4 trillion per year due to increased life expectancy.

One other very significant problem that drives Big Pharma, enabling them to create medication that can be harmful, is our misplaced sense of trust of any industry that we believe has a record of safety. The processed food and automobile industries are good examples. From your point of view—the person who is taking a medication and wants to make sure it is safe, you might think that the more often a certain drug is used, there is less danger. For example *50 billion aspirin tablets* are consumed worldwide each year with mostly justified expectations that it will help heart patients with anticlotting effects and reduce fevers.

Despite its relatively positive history, aspirin can be a dangerous drug, interacting with other drugs, and sometimes provoking severe gastric side effects. No one has called for this Big Pharma money maker to be banned. Today, because of its anticlotting properties and potential for interactions, aspirin might be a prescription drug when introduced into the market. This is a classic example of why you have to be careful with "safe drugs". Ironically, both cocaine and marijuana have been easily available, legal and considered effective, multiple times in the 20th century. Cocaine was literally an ingredient in Coca Cola and marijuana, in its "hemp-rope-like" form has been grown for more than 12,000 years and was legal until the early 1900's and is back again, marketed as "medical marijuana."

OUR HEALTH AND MEDICATION:

The latest report shows continued improvements in the health of Americans, with life expectancy at birth up to 77.3 years in 2002, a record, and deaths from heart disease, cancer and stroke – the nation's three leading killers – all down 1 percent to 3 percent.

Adult use of antidepressants almost tripled between 1988-1994 and 1999-2000. Ten percent of women 18 and older and 4 percent of men now take antidepressants. Prescriptions for nonsteroidal anti-inflammatory drugs, antidepressants, blood glucose/sugar regulators, and cholesterol-lowering statin drugs, in particular, increased notably between 1996 and 2002.

The National Health and Nutrition Examination Survey found a 13 percent increase between 1988-1994 and 1999-2000 in the proportion of Americans taking at least one drug and a 40 percent jump in the proportion taking three or more medicines. Forty-four percent reported taking at least one drug in the past month and 17 percent were taking three or more in the 2000 survey.

The annual report to Congress showed that health expenditures climbed 9.3 percent in 2002 to $1.6 trillion. Although prescription drugs comprise only one-tenth of the total medical bill, they remain the fastest growing expenditure. The price of drugs rose 5 percent, but wider use of medicines pushed total expenditures up 15.3 percent in 2002.

Drug expenditures have risen at least 15 percent every year since 1998.

Who Created "The Market" (Or Who Made The First Pill?)

As a "consumer" of pills, there are many reasons to have a working knowledge of the history of medications, how they were developed, and the context. Since almost everyone uses medicines, understanding the reason for their development can help you identify when a drug is not working and when there is potential interaction danger from use of other medication that your physician has not asked about.

Modern medications, those we use as a primary treatment for virtually any disease, have a sort of rollercoaster history. Many evolved thousands of years ago to treat various illnesses (i.e. infections) that were mysterious and virulent. Others had been used successfully for generations, but were banned for newly evolving religious and superstitious reasons. Some of this was partly rational since many were ineffective.

Seen from today's pharmacopoeia of miracle medicines, many treatments of the past made no sense, were barbaric and of little value. The medicines that did develop were based on everything from "textbooks" written on papyrus to myths and legends passed down from each generation. Geography, religion, deification of magicians (remember Merlin?) kept the development of effective medicines from progressing too rapidly. Roadblocks caused by wars, plagues and other disasters wiped out significant progress, but led to newer ideas and the extraordinary successes that we've seen in the last 125 years from the turn of the century, WWI, WWII, Korea, Vietnam to Afghanistan.

With the exception of many Asian and Middle Eastern civilizations, our own arrogance has contributed to drug abuse by refusing to consider "alternative medications" and supplements. Our historical path of medical treatments has often been considered of no value to succeeding generations—until today's more enlightened attitude. Alternative medications, supplements and herbal treatments were not even studied scientifically by researchers at the National Institutes of Health until the past decade.

It is not all bad news since development of effective medication has closely followed the success of medical practice itself. There have been dedicated physicians and scientists, working in large companies and also people in basement labs seeking answers to perplexing health disasters. Most of the great breakthroughs have been *need driven,* but the discovery that unintended "pleasurable" side-effects created feelings that seemed at the time to be a "bonus", turned out to be a disaster. This drive to find cures does often result in addiction no matter how legitimate the goal would seem to be, or, even more likely, the source of the advice. Would you say no to Sigmund Freud when he told you all your personal problems would vanish with a sniff of this white powder even though it was cocaine and legal?

The Timeline of Addiction

There have been at least eight to ten distinct phases in the development of medications that represent the advancing nature of the most significant societies. All of them have, in one way or another, produced seemingly benign effects, but ended up damaging some of the people who were initially helped. Unfortunately the knowledge did not spread as much as it could have and copious documents were lost. The spread of medical knowledge and useful medicines did not really develop until global travel became possible and cultures became more sophisticated. Adventurers, like the renowned Marco

Polo and explorers from the England and Spain seeking precious gems, colonized medically sophisticated countries like India (or South America) and returned with medical bounties greater than gold. Ironically, one prized treasure was tobacco, a product that fits the model above as a good discovery turning out very badly. The major cultures that ultimately led us to where we are now include:

- Egypt (5000-3000 BC)

- Mesopotamia—Babylon (2nd Millennium)

- India & Asia (600 BC—ongoing)

- China (5th century BC--ongoing)

- Greece & Rome (700 BC)

- Islamic Society/Persia (ongoing)

- The Middle Ages (1100-16th Century)

- Renaissance to Early Modern (17th Century)

- Modern—18th Century (ongoing)

Egypt: The Real Cradle of Medicine

We might know more than we do now if some of the advanced, ancient societies' understanding of the body and how it functions had survived longer. Early civilizations like the Egyptians are a prime example and were more advanced than one might think. Their medical development led to a very interesting, true version of the roots of today's health care system.

Various sources going back as far as 3000 BC, documented that the Egyptians, while still using some mystic incantations also recognized that public health was part of keeping the population alive. The Egyptians were among the first, along with other Middle Eastern civilizations, to recognize that some of the types of food, sexual behavior, and excess drinking were part of a negative lifestyle. As organized governments and communities emerged in the Middle East, they became responsible for enforcing these policies and their overall health and lifespan increased.

For many civilizations pain killing was a primary goal and Egypt was no exception. There are records that indicate that as far back as 2000 B.C. opium was commonly used to treat everything from tooth pain to headaches. It was often combined with wine and used as a children's sedative, a teething remedy, and to achieve a state of calm. Several accounts of medicine in ancient Egypt pointed out that many "healers" specialized in a single disease, and now, 3000 years later we have a similar system. Fortunately, there was lucky event that did give us a clear idea of how advanced the Middle Eastern approach to medication had become. We were aware that surgical procedures were being used, although the sophistication of the ancients was not fully recognized until the mid 1860's. An American antiquities dealer, Edwin Smith, stumbled upon a book or "papyrus" (an early version of paper created by the stems of the papyrus plant harvested in marshes). Coincidentally, the antique shop happened to be in Luxor, Egypt— the capital of ancient Egypt and the location of many historic temples and shrines. Smith, recognizing that this could be a 2500 year old medical text book, began translating and discovered that it was essentially a series of medical "case notes" exactly the way we keep medical records today.

The Egyptians' and other ancient civilizations' understanding of the body and how to repair it was quite surprising, especially considering what came afterwards.

For example:

- The earliest reported surgery was performed in Egypt around 2750 BC.

- Head injuries along with neck, arms, lips, throat, the shoulder and torso were also described along with directions for using stitches to close the wounds with sutures.

- The practice of immobilizing someone who may have a neck or back injury was also practiced and is still a standard practice by EMT's who arrive at an accident and are trying to stabilize a victim.

- One of the most interesting aspects of these documents is that they describe the cranial <u>structures</u>, the anatomy of the central nervous system, brain anatomy, certain aspects of the blood flow system in and around the brain, and how various organs function.

- It is possible that the first pill came about sometime during this era as Egypt's continued understanding of physiology grew. It is also possible that the "pill" was simply a powdered medicine wrapped in a leaf to make it easier to swallow—in other words, the pill is a delivery system.

The bad news about this extraordinary civilization is that it eventually followed a road that was going to be more common in the future for all countries. According to a report by Narcon International, a drug rehab group that has a facility in Egypt:

> *The ancient culture of Egypt includes an equally ancient history of drug and alcohol abuse. Opium and hashish have been used in Egypt for centuries, and recent tests have found cocaine in mummified remains - a discovery that has confounded historians who considered that the coca plant was purely a South American phenomenon until recent times.*
>
> *It was in the 1980s that use of narcotics began to escalate to serious levels. Currently, Egypt is one of Africa's top cultivators of cannabis and opium poppies. The number of hectares discovered that are dedicated to growing addictive substances have been increasing steadily over the last decade. The amount of "bango" - the local name for marijuana - seizures has also been increasing from 60,000 kg per year up to 80,000 kg and above. In addition to cultivation, opium and heroin are transported in from Southwest and Southeast Asia*
>
> *It is estimated that addicts in Egypt are spending $2.9 billion on drugs each year. Estimates on how many people are addicted to opiates, cannabis, amphetamine-type stimulants or heroin vary greatly, but range between 600,000 and 800,000, according to a 2007 study.*
>
> *Half the 129,850 people who entered drug rehabs in 2007 were addicted to cannabis, while another 43 percent were dependent on opiates of various types. Another 7 percent were addicts of amphetamine-type stimulants that would include ecstasy and methamphetamine, sniffing, cannabis or prescription drug abuse.*

For those with more income, alcohol, cocaine, heroin, cannabis, ecstasy and methamphetamine are regularly abused. More than 12 percent of Egyptian students are dependent on drugs and another 9 percent to bango and 3 percent to hashish.

In 2005, the total number of heroin addicts in Egypt were estimated to run somewhere between 20,000 and 30,000. A 2007 report stated that 8.5 percent of Egyptians -or six million people -are addicted to drugs. The majority of them are between 15 and 25 years of age.

Greece & Rome: Evolution

Over the next several thousand years, well into the era of the Greek and Roman empires, medicine and medications as powders or potions continued to evolve. Around 460 BC, the Greek physician, Hippocrates was born and later emerged as one of the few physicians who believed that illness was rooted in physical causes, not evil spirits lurking about. He documented symptoms of pneumonia and epilepsy in children and theorized that people recovered from illness quicker if their attitude was positive. In fact his approach today would be called "holistic" and he believed in treating the whole body—not parts. In effect, Hippocrates recognized that there were connections between diseases and he detailed these ideas in his tests that influenced medicine for two centuries after his death. In his records he mentions a juice called *mecon* with both anti-purgative and narcotic action. However, the *meconion* of Greek botanist, Theophrastus (372-287 BC), is the first authentic reference to the juice of the poppy.

This was a low moment for the drug addiction plague—perhaps Egypt was more than The Cradle of Civilization.

According to Dr. Anil Aggrawal, in his book *Narcotic Drugs*, he indicates that,

The Greek poet, Homer (9th century BC) was aware of opium and mentions it in his epics *Iliad* and *Odyssey*. In his time the use of a peculiar drug, Nepenthes, also known as the 'drug of forgetfulness', was fairly widespread in Greece. Opium was a major constituent of Nepenthes. It also appears that Greek warriors regularly took Nepenthes before going to war in order to dull their senses to danger.

Rome was also developing a reasonably civilized society and medical system with sewers and a banking system. It was clear to the Romans that waste disposal was critical to public health. Unfortunately, for the three centuries before the fall of Rome, its one million inhabitants were under the control of maniacal emperors like Nero, who destabilized any real progress. As Rome devolved over the next 1000 years, many of the public health practices and enlightened teachings disappeared and tribal life ruled once again.

The Decline of The Roman-Opiate Empire

Galen was the foremost physician in Rome from about AD 169-192. It was Galen who so enthusiastically lauded the virtues of opium that its popularity grew to new heights by the end of the second century. The drug was even distributed by Roman shopkeepers and itinerant quacks, following its release for common use by Roman Emperor, Severus, at the end of the second century.

From this time on, the evolution of medicine sank from the progressive approach of the ancients to a period of mystery, misinformation, mysticism, wizardry, and religious fear. Through this era, known now as medieval times, or the Dark Ages and the Middle Ages, medicine became little more than a series of incantations and superstitions.

China, Japan, Asia: Medicine Goes Global

Only Asian countries such as China and Japan (also India) made any significant progress in healing during these periods; however, they were largely cut off from the Western civilizations and also suffered from internal warfare. The Chinese did, as early as 1000 BC, create a form of inoculation that could lead to immunity and could protect children from smallpox. Of course, there are also countless mentions of opium in the travel histories from the 9th Century on that included most of the eastern Asian and Mediterranean countries.

Modern medication in China may also be responsible for an early form of "pills" that were part of what has became a very large business—patent medicines. Usually these were a combination of herbs, dried and turned into a powder, formed into pills and in China many ended up rolled into a shiny black ball called the Black

Pearl. But that was China where virtually everything from silk to gunpowder, rockets (and fireworks) printing, paper and even the compass was invented.

Across Europe most of the population was now illiterate—kept that way by the church. Books were discarded and medical science gave way to overbearing religious beliefs. Alcohol and opium, of course, were widely used as the only forms of "anesthesia" or neuralgia along with mandrake for virtually all problems from wounds to gout and as a "passion potion." Hemlock was used for everything, but had serious side effects including death. Opium, alcohol, and other opiates became medical staples and continued for hundreds of years—especially on the European continent.

The Dark Ages/Medieval Times

During the Dark Ages the responsibility of directly curing any medical problem was mostly a function of the church priests. This attitude characterized any problem as a sign that you had angered God and prayer might (but usually did not) help. It is more likely that the total lack of hygiene hastened more deaths and spread plagues both in Europe and in conquered lands such as North and South America.

The Dark Ages were not without any "health care system," but in this case they were monasteries founded by St. Benedict—a monk who devoted himself and the Benedictine followers who dedicated their lives to helping the sick. Despite their efforts and kindness, unfortunately their approach was simply to pray and establish shrines that would either cure someone—or not. Survival, they also felt, was God's will.

Opium however was still around and widely used. A form called laudanum appeared in the 17th Century for dysentery. It became the medicine/drug of choice for famous British poets because it was the perfect drug for everything: 10% opium, 1gm of morphine and topped off by alcohol.

Over the centuries society's approach to health and healing slowly disentangled itself from the overwhelming grip of various religions. New approaches to medicine have enabled us to connect one disease to another. If it were not for two specific, but surprising events, we might still be brewing root teas and waving palm leaves over people with heart attacks.

One significant change and an obvious one was the rise of the public health movement and the other was, ironically, the "benefits" of war.

By the early 17th and 18th centuries, central governments had established themselves across the globe and literacy spread even though the religious orders kept control in many places. The government leaders began to realize that without some sort of public health "policies" that would maintain order, disease would continue to spread and overwhelm those trying to change the general lack of interest in good health. This problem exists today with "fat cities", nationwide diet programs, and focus on the massive outbreaks of diabetes and obesity. However, in the United States, very little focus has been in this direction until the rise of public health nursing and child welfare services in the 1930's.

As you can see from the brief recap above, the use of medications over the millennia has literally been a process to climb one hill, go around a roadblock and be persistent. Ironically, today we've ended up with some of the medical practices that date back to Ancient Egypt when a "specialist," a practice that is still strong, treated you. Ironically there is one more aspect of medical and human history that has created great change and promises to bring more that will even affect the cardio-diabetes connection.

Medicine (And Addiction) Comes To America:

It is likely that the use of most medications (usually some sort of opiate or alcohol) in North America followed or accompanied the British colonists who arrived on our shores in the 16th and 17th Centuries. During that time in the U.K., the British had begun a campaign to reduce the phony healers who dispensed patent medication—both as pills and liquids. While reducing the number of fakes, it led to another medication called Morrison's Pill.

The theory of Morrison's Pill, it seems, was to "cleanse the body" and many of these were laxatives. *The irony is that these drugs became the first abused drugs.* Often "patients" took dozens of pills with the intention to clean out their system totally. Unfortunately many had a stronger than "normal" result. Not only was this one-size-fits-all medicine soon sold around the world, but the directions for use were along the lines of "as many as you wish." This led to an odd addiction that does create a weird visual so ultimately, the British passed laws regulating medicine more closely. This is yet another clear example that a positive a drug's intention can be a debacle; and the human element is the key that gets turned on to start the process.

Conceptually, patent medicines were a good idea since it was intended to lead to an industry of regulation. Unfortunately as the U.S. grew, its medical and health needs demanded something that was good for any ailment; the old "quick fix." Few of these drugs were ever really patented (some patented the bottles) and many of the ingredients were the same—and useless. Heavily promoted in ads and direct sales on the street, (as shown in the movies) literally thousands of patent medicines appeared at the same time Chinese and English products were imported in the beginning of the 17th Century, driving US sales.

This is probably when our nascent "pharmaceutical industry" became an addiction enabler. The main ingredients for most of these was, perhaps a ground vegetable base (for flavor) followed by strong alcohol, some morphine, a dose of opium topped off with cocaine. Sounds like it can't fail to at least make someone "better" for a while. Unfortunately people of all ages, including children were regular users.

If you look back at the descriptions of addiction in Chapter One they included compulsive use despite the consequences. The patent medication industry actually launched the pharmaceutical industry and addiction rehab business at one time with a single product to cure everything. Only the labels changed.

By the way, it was not long before large catalog companies like Sears sold specialized products for children. One called "Soothing Baby Syrup" did the job—it was laced with morphine creating a stoned (but quiet) toddler.

Our first real significant contribution to the development of medication (and addiction) was, most likely before and after the Civil War. Sadly, this follows the historical paths of many other cultures— war helps new medicine and medication development, but the cost may be many lives to "try different methods". The Civil War was known for its amputations (three out of every four operations were amputations) and survivors who lived in pain and on addictive opiates. Today there remain very active surgeons groups who dispute whether or not many of these radical and crude amputations were necessary.

During the war and soon after, the first pharmacies (called apothecaries for centuries) appeared in colonial villages where medicine may have been dispensed as powder in hand-crafted, easy to take "pills". We do know from a variety of records that the North used more than one million pain pills—either morphine or an opiate of some kind during treatment for wounds.

1700-1930: The Alcoholic Republic:

There has always been another drug used for self-medication, but really not seen as one. Of course; that is alcohol. It is important to keep in mind that drinking was one of the most important pastimes over two centuries. Most people in our large cities filled the pubs or bars after work and established a pattern of "use" that matches our modern definition of addiction—and easy access as noted above for burgeoning alcohol addicts. How many times have you heard or said "I'll just have one." Again, supply and demand. In the more rural areas there were roadhouses where travelers stopped (most people traveled by horseback well into the mid-1800's.) These were the precursors of today's motels, but usually with a dining room/bar that served little to drink beyond beer and wine brewed locally, often by the monks in the local church—who also ran things in town.

The amount of alcohol, consumed by the average person not only gave rise to the nickname The Alcoholic Republic, but also created a whole new industry. Sometimes called the "drunk tank," later "asylums for the inebriated" and then "rehab" where many alcoholic relatives frequently disappeared.

Even though patent medicines with strong alcohol bases remain on the market today, legitimate doctors and pharmacists have fought them, recognizing they were ineffective and potentially harmful. The battle to ban them (or regulate the ingredients) continued throughout the 19th Century until political movements, especially the temperance movement who were against anything that contained alcohol, reduced the size of the industry.

Eventually in the 19th Century, pharmacy developed into a serious academic and regulated profession. Many drugs were

created by compounding (the reason why th
a pharmacy symbol) and this evolved into ɟ
doses. Digoxin for the heart and high bloo
are typical examples that developed in the lat
remain in our formulary.

Interestingly, for some around the turn (
and cocaine were available and it is estimated t
addicts.

Modern Medication: The

The 20th Century was an era of serious regul;
of real scientific study of the efficacy of medic;
Food and Drug Act. Two forces played signific
or controlling patent medicines: President Ted
a fanatic conservationist and Upton Sinclair, th
who wrote an exposé of the horrific condition
industry. By 1906 the legislation to launch t
became the Food and Drug Administration
Congress. This widespread movement, with
tagged Muckrakers, had reported on sickened
during the Spanish-American War and succee
backing.

The FDA act also required prescriptions
a legitimate doctor and that all potentially
labeled. The FDA now began supervising tes
medication for everyone. Not surprisingly, lob
drug industry descended on Washington, but

One thing to note is that currently pate
form of herbs, supplements and vitamins are
drug store, health food store and supermark
remain, "*This statement has not been evaluated
Administration. This product is not intended to
prevent any disease.*" The rationale is that these
supplements and are not advertised as a medic

Me

I
have
100
plag
in th
that

"sna
Big I
majc
Phar
press
the
gove
enga

wars
Wars
Afgh
odd
limb
this.
deve
supp

med
befo
from
knov
bad
heal
anyc
and
heal
STE

icine Enters the Future: Good News & Bad

is very hard to over-emphasize the changes in our lives that
been created by drugs and medical breakthroughs in the past
ears. From the beginning of the 20th Century and into the 21st,
s, global disease and super-medications that can target places
brain and calm the troubled are just a small slice of a picture
as both a positive and negative side.

day an industry that began as mom and pop operations selling
oil" has turned into a gigantic group of conglomerates (aka
harma) that, collectively earn $315 billion a year. Most of the
drug companies today got their start with patent medicines.
acists or doctors opened storefront dispensaries with pill
ng devices or mixing bowls for liquids. Selling directly to
nsumer, a new industry without any interference from any
ment agency developed where one could make any claim and
e in drug making without any credentials.

The 20th Century And War:

e effects of medicine and substance abuse during the various
of the 20th Century are profound. This includes the two World
Korea, Vietnam and the three most recent wars in Kuwait,
nistan, and Iraq. Perhaps the easiest way to evaluate it is an
actoid; over the years there have been more "wounded and
lost" and fewer fatalities. There are TWO basic reasons for
his is a clear demonstration of the guiding principle of medical
pment; the classic combination of science and the law of
y and demand.

any World War I (WWI) related breakthroughs are obvious—
ations—antibiotics and others for wound care were developed
e and after WWI. Still, after that war 20 million people died
what was thought to be a flu epidemic in Britain. Now we
it had nothing to do with war or a plague. Rather it was simple
ygiene, especially among the poor. A drive to increase public
began and by the time of WWII antibiotics were available to
e— especially the Armed Forces. This lesson stuck in the U.K.
1948, after WWII the U.K. established permanent national
care to deal with both wounded soldiers and high rates of
s.

In general, the "drug of choice" by both the U.K. and the Germans in WWI was alcohol and daily rations of rum or beer were made available in most of their wars. Drug use in WW II and Vietnam is also well documented:

In WWII, the German army seemed to exist on methamphetamine to keep soldiers alert and functional for several hours/days—especially because rations were minimal. Records show that 35 million tablets of methamphetamine were shipped to the army and air force between just April and July 1940 alone. Even though they were banned, another 10 million were eventually distributed to soldiers.

The use of alcohol was also encouraged by the German military. Alcohol became a crutch for many of the men serving at the time. This prevalent and habitual use of alcohol led to many otherwise preventable deaths and injuries. Production of bootlegged alcohol became a serious issue, as many producers didn't know the difference between consumable alcohol and methyl-alcohol. Men who consumed spirits made with methyl-alcohol became blind or succumbed to fatal alcohol poisoning.

World War II and Korea saw the level of wounded rise, but this time; there were no breakthrough medications. However, the development of technology such as advanced X-rays and the electron microscope helped understand the body. What has been the secret seemed to be quickly airlifting the wounded back behind lines and stabilizing them. Remember the visual of choppers; swooping in under heavy gunfire in M.A.S.H. and Vietnam to airlift the "grunts?"

Vietnam might have been our first war where recreational medication played a role. As we now know, that part of the world was a major drug import and production junction.

If you've seen one movie about 'Nam' you know that pot was the number one drug. It is one thing to fight a war drunk or on speed — but not stoned. The Army tried policing the situation and when finally, arrests rose to 1,000 per week, the Army was so concerned that they began massive treatment and interdiction programs. However, in retrospect apparently the soldiers policed their own, making sure that their own men were sober enough to be effective on the battlefield.

The military was also concerned about opiates such as heroin and cocaine that were produced in the so-called **Golden Triangle** where most of Asia's two opium-producing areas were located. Much of the information about it is sketchy and reported to be an area of around 367,000 square miles (950,000 km^2) that overlaps the mountains of four countries of Southeast Asia: Burma, Vietnam, Laos, and Thailand.

Today Afghanistan and Pakistan, along with their corrupt leaders, have so much saturation of opiate "dirt" that much of their populations, including children, are hooked. Beginning in the 1920's the production of heroin was mostly in the old Golden Triangle but Pakistan and Afghanistan now run the worldwide show.

The recent wars in the Middle East brought a new challenge. A system was designed to have "forward quick" ERs designed to be near the battles' forward lines. Anyone wounded could be stabilized quickly and then flown to major surgical centers in Germany or elsewhere. There have been at least 723 casualties who have required amputations but now many do recover with artificial limbs and physical therapy.

More Soldiers Are Saved—More Opiates Abused

Today's military has changed the paradigm for lowering amputations, but strong pain killers are still a problem and many families don't recognize either the problems or symptoms like drinking or PTSD. According to the National Institutes of Health,

> *Over the past 56 months, of the 8058 military casualties meeting the listed criteria, 5684 (70.5%) were recorded as having major limb injuries. Of these, 423 (5.2% of all serious injuries; 7.4% of major limb injuries) underwent major limb amputation or amputation at or proximal to the wrist or ankle joint. The mechanism of injury for 87.9% was some form of explosive device. The major amputation rate during Vietnam was 8.3% of major limb injuries. Overall, major limb amputation rates for the current*
> *U.S. engagement in Afghanistan and Iraq are similar to those of previous conflicts.*

Medication, however has played a strong role in assisting the wounded from recent strife, although very little hard information is now available on substance abuse other than psychiatric drugs that seem to be widely abused. Suicides and major mental illness plus addiction and alcoholism have become common and government agencies like the VA who are supposed to take responsibility for this have had their funding slashed.

Perhaps the worst aspect of the current wars in Afghanistan and Iraq is that we've created an entire new "branch of medicine" for pain and mental health problems from the appearance of widespread post traumatic stress disorder (PTSD). There are thousands of wounded Middle East veteran soldiers, many in their early 20's with injuries that have cost them multiple limbs. For them, their entire lives and futures will forever be a major challenge.

Unfortunately, the pain that occurs with war wounds is severe and the drugs of choice are oxycodone and hydrocodone, both of which are highly addictive. These young soldiers have been dropped into a *perfect storm* and set up for addiction. While we have attempted to manage their pain or emotional problems, the rate of suicides among our military is not only the highest since records have been taken but higher than the rate among civilians. Ironically, all our soldiers are given psych evaluations before entering the service but not necessarily when redeployed—and many return for multiple tours.

Big Pharma Today:

By the 1960's, the standard for approval of a drug was not simply that it worked, but was safe. This had a significant effect on medications here but even more directly on imported meds that had not undergone the same rigorous testing required in the U.S. This has not always worked and below are some examples of medication— often developed for one disorder that proves either lethal or addicting or can be said to be safe. (i.e. thalidomide on the down side and erectile dysfunction medications on the up).

In many ways it is easiest to look at drug development through the actions or motivations of the researchers or scientists whose focus may have been on a small sample of an herb or a synthetic substance— even taking chances testing it on themselves. It is also obvious, if you watch TV, that the number of ads for pills to solve a problem no matter how private it is are ubiquitous. The battles between the drug companies have led to high research and development costs that have been passed onto everyone—not just those who need a pill once a year.

Drug companies have only 20 years to protect their investment with a copyright. Then the drugs go off of brand name protection and are sold as generics, much below the former retail costs (and less stringent tests). Prices for generics can be 10% of the former cost. Many people try to mail order medication from outside the U.S. Be aware that these can frequently be dangerous and are prepared under less regulated circumstances.

Chapter Four

Why Certain "Medications" Have Become "Recreational Drugs" Today.

Medications developed across the ages were never *designed* to be "fun or recreational." In almost every case where a drug became part of the culture of abuse, it was first hailed as a "miracle" and a significant number actually have changed our world permanently. Many of these breakthrough drugs like pain killers (opiates) that have been used for centuries ultimately harmed people, but were not illegal—at first. Some, due to continued use in different cultures (cannabis), were simply "legal" by default. Others have been widely used until the laws changed as the physical toll became obvious. Unfortunately there always seems to be a loophole to slip through to a waiting potential addict or abuser.

This pattern of learning "too-late" about the dangers of a medication is consistent over generations whether the drug has potential for addiction or simply serious hidden side effects that only emerge as significant after larger numbers of patients have used them. We've mentioned a few like thalidomide, but others like guaranteed weight loss solutions and drugs to treat cancer that proved ineffective (exotic supplements and herbs) appear more frequently, as "similar over-the-counter compounds" than you would think. This loop is repeated frequently and is an often overlooked reason why many new drugs of abuse, like different versions of anti-anxiety medications, appear and are sold illicitly and often at great profit despite regulation.

One of the most disturbing aspects of drug use today is clear in the statistics that follow and describe adolescent drug use—a problem that's widely recognized, but with only one real solution: prevention. Of course this is a simplistic approach because the various educational programs in schools or private programs have failed to significantly reduce use of every drug from marijuana to prescription drugs and over-the-counter cough medicine.

Is There An Answer For This Problem?

There are numerous programs or guides instructing parents how to recognize the signs and behavior of a kid on drugs. Most of these are obvious such as dropping grades, new friends, odd behavior or loss of interest in their major activities. However, you've done what you shouldn't do. For example, you've searched Billy's drawers, read Suzie's diary, or even had hair from their brush sent to a lab for testing, yet found nothing.

You've overlooked one thing. Teenagers are, as you probably were, very good at keeping parents in the dark. As odd as this may sound you have missed one part of their lives that you can't see— what are they listening to. Think back to the late 1950's. What was your parent's reaction to Elvis and why? Easy one. They saw swiveled hipped sex but you saw this great looking guy with great music to dance to. Or later into the 1960's when Van Morrison sang about his "Brown Eyed Girl". For the boomers, Van was talking about love, but now many say the BEG was really heroin. Another good example is The Eagles' "Hotel California" or literally hundreds of hits by the other obvious groups like the Stones and The Doors. The drug references in the past few decades were also part of the culture including folkies like John Denver ("…lie there with my old lady and pass the pipe around…")

Today your kid has a very wide choice in music and a specific choice that we did not have. Like all music, each generation owns its songs but now many of the popular rap songs, are openly violent and like Eminem's "Little Purple Pills" make no effort to disguise their point.

The bottom line is this: Don't simply rely on visible evidence in regard to your adolescents and drug abuse. Look at their cultural interests; in the boomers history, the Beatles are a prime example. While there are drug references in their music, the Beatles wrote about peace and love and their music lives on. Today, guns and macho posing may be the message your child is listening to on their iPod.

"Good Drugs" Go Bad: The 20th Century

One reason so many basically useless or dangerous medications came on the market from the 18th Century on is the evolution of our belief in "experts" who usually have only the best intentions. The role played in the various medieval societies by "apothecaries" has been an influential part of today's evolving healthcare system (even partially stretching back to biblical times). These precursors to modern pharmacists played a significant role in the perception of the safety of many medications—and given the low level of scientific knowledge by the public at that time—was not unjustified.

Over centuries medications came from two sources:

- The local "apothecary" who was regarded as a skilled and educated individual who made the medications and also gave out (costly) medical advice.

- Experienced midwifes or, more likely various orders of nuns who assisted with births and "female problems."

The dominance of this system in the 15th and 16th Century was often tied to religious orders with a monopoly on the market, secured by a relationship with the "Royals." On the other hand, many peasants were given crude medications like a **poultice** whose ingredients changed depending on whose recipe was being used—sort of an early version of the "house special". The willing acceptance of the people who were grateful for any help advanced the idea that anything from an "official" was embraced.

This attitude carried on and by the 18th and 19th Centuries, retail shops and the new apothecaries (now called pharmacists) were developing a much more professional and restricted approach to dispensing medicine. Still, obtaining dangerous drugs like opiates in privately run opium dens found globally in the Victorian era was relatively simple.

"O Romeo, Romeo! Wherefore art thou Romeo?"

One famous mention of an apothecary was made by William Shakespeare in *Romeo and Juliet*, in which a "poor apothecary" sells Romeo an elixir of death with which Romeo commits suicide. This is actually a fascinating historical precursor of the use of a medication created by a trusted "professional" person to overdose since both Romeo and the apothecary were well aware of this effect of the drug.

What It's Like In The Trenches:

Before looking at how many totally legal, not to mention effective medications, became widespread drugs of abuse, consider the results of a yearly survey conducted by the Substance Abuse and Mental Health Services Administration (SAMHSA) mentioned in the Introduction. The study covers use among young children, adolescents, and adults of both genders. It's important to keep in mind that the results of this study and many others show that the earlier someone begins drug abuse the more likely they are to continue. Please note that 'past month' in the statistics below refer to the previous month before taking the survey.

Here are a few very disturbing highlights of the SAMHSA report:

- In 2009, an estimated 21.8 million Americans aged 12 or older were current (past month) illicit drug users. This estimate represents 8.7 percent of the population aged 12 or older. Illicit drugs include marijuana/hashish, cocaine (including crack), heroin, hallucinogens, inhalants, or prescription-type psychotherapeutics used nonmedically.

- The rate of current illicit drug use among persons aged 12 or older in 2009 (8.7 percent) was higher than the rate in 2008 (8.0 percent).

- In 2009, there were 1.6 million current cocaine users aged 12 or older, comprising 0.7 percent of the population. These estimates were similar to the number and rate in 2008 (1.9 million or 0.7 percent) but were lower than the estimates in 2006 (2.4 million or 1.0 percent).

- Hallucinogens were used in the past month by 1.3 million persons (0.5 percent) aged 12 or older in 2009, including 760,000 (0.3 percent) who had used Ecstasy. The number and percentage of Ecstasy users increased between 2008 (555,000 or 0.2 percent) and 2009.

- In 2009, there were 7.0 million (2.8 percent) persons aged 12 or older who used prescription- type psychotherapeutic drugs nonmedically in the past month. These estimates were higher than in 2008 (6.2 million or 2.5 percent), but similar to estimates in 2007 (6.9 million or 2.8 percent).

- The number of past month methamphetamine users decreased between 2006 and 2008, but then increased in 2009. The numbers were 731,000 (0.3 percent) in 2006, 529,000 (0.2 percent) in 2007, 314,000 (0.1 percent) in 2008, and 502,000 (0.2 percent) in 2009.

- Among youths aged 12 to 17, the current illicit drug use rate increased from 2008 (9.3 percent) to 2009 (10.0 percent). Between 2002 and 2008, the rate declined from 11.6 to 9.3 percent.

- Among youths aged 12 to 17, the rate of nonmedical use of prescription-type drugs declined from 4.0 percent in 2002 to 2.9 percent in 2008, then held steady at 3.1 percent in 2009.

- The rate of current Ecstasy use among youths aged 12 to 17 declined from 0.5 percent in 2002 to 0.3 percent in 2004, remained at that level through 2007, and then increased to 0.5 percent in 2009.

- Between 2008 and 2009, the rate of current use of illicit drugs among young adults aged 18 to 25 increased from 19.6 to 21.2 percent, driven largely by an increase in marijuana use (from 16.5 to 18.1 percent).

- From 2002 to 2009, there was an increase among young adults aged 18 to 25 in the rate of current nonmedical use of prescription-type drugs (from 5.5 to 6.3 percent), driven primarily by an increase in pain reliever misuse (from 4.1 to 4.8 percent). There were decreases in the use of cocaine (from 2.0 to 1.4 percent) and methamphetamine (from 0.6 to 0.2 percent).

- Among those aged 50 to 59, the rate of past month illicit drug use increased from 2.7 percent in 2002 to 6.2 percent in 2009. This trend partially reflects the aging entry into this age group of the baby boom cohort, whose lifetime rate of illicit drug use is higher than those of older cohorts.

- Among persons aged 12 or older in 2008-2009 who used pain relievers nonmedically in the past 12 months, 55.3 percent got the drug they most recently used from a friend or relative for free. Another 17.6 percent reported they got the drug from one doctor. Only 4.8 percent got pain relievers from a drug dealer or other stranger, and 0.4 percent bought them on the Internet. Among those who reported getting the pain reliever from a friend or relative for free, 80.0 percent reported in a follow-up question that the friend or relative had obtained the drugs from just one doctor.

- Among unemployed adults aged 18 or older in 2009, 17.0 percent were current illicit drug users, which was higher than the 8.0 percent of those employed full time and 11.5 percent of those employed part time. However, most illicit drug users were employed. Of the 19.3 million current illicit drug users aged 18 or older in 2009, 12.9 million (66.6 percent) were employed either full or part time. The number of unemployed illicit drug users increased from 1.3 million in 2007 to 1.8 million in 2008 and 2.5 million in 2009, primarily because of an overall increase in the number of unemployed persons.

- In 2009, 10.5 million persons aged 12 or older reported driving under the influence of illicit drugs during the past year. This corresponds to 4.2 percent of the population aged 12 or older, which is similar to the rate in 2008 (4.0 percent) and the rate in 2002 (4.7 percent). In 2009, the rate was highest among young adults aged 18 to 25 (12.8 percent).

Marijuana: From Hemp To The Bong: The Most Abused Drug Today

There is no substance that can better illustrate the lessons of a drug perceived to be safe, but "gone bad" than the hyper-fertile cannabis plant once found almost everywhere and was widely used by anyone for eons. *This plant, mostly known as "weed" tops the list of drugs of abuse that have been illegal for less than a century but were also legal and valuable for as far back as recorded history has uncovered.* This is the essential problem that marijuana and other drugs can create where safety and addiction is concerned.

There is no question that it seems strange today that a product of this plant called **hemp,** was used to make high quality "canvas" sails in the Revolutionary War for ships like Old Ironsides. Not only would it become illegal but now tops the charts, ranked as a totally banned and most dangerous drug.

Ironically, today, after tobacco, marijuana is still the most commonly smoked drug yet tobacco is essentially legal and available everywhere.

Hemp

The conundrum is not as puzzling as it may seem. Until the 20th Century cannabis (a.k.a marijuana) was quite valuable as a source of the fibers for hemp that could be also used around the plantation for many products from clothing to rope. Few, if any growers knew much about its psychoactive properties or the fact that only one strain would eventually be more valuable as a commodity than something to mellow out with after a long day in the fields.

The Marijuana "Twins": Behind The High

Marijuana or **cannabis** is a very sturdy, fast growing plant that has mostly been used for many industrial purposes. Few understand that there are really two different strains of cannabis, a male and a female that look very similar and are both banned despite their disparate histories, use and the "high" they deliver.

If the ancient Egyptians or the colonial settlers were to visit us in the 21st Century and drop into a department store to buy a coat or dress, they would probably wonder why the fibers used to make its product and material were now some sort of synthetic. It's more than likely they'd ask, "Where are the good hemp clothes?" While our time travelers may have known a little about today's dangerous female marijuana they may not have thought much about it. They called the actual plant Cannabis Sativa (Latin for planted hemp) and discovered that its fiber was as strong as cotton for making clothes and ropes for ships—vital elements in that pre-industrial period.

Marijuana or cannabis also has a unique agricultural history and has been found in so many places because it is known to grow quickly and was thought to have a variety of other medicinal uses. It also developed an odd distinction during Colonial America. Ironically all farmers were actually required by law in Jamestown VA, (1619) to grow hemp or be jailed. It could even be used as a substitute for money—accepted by merchants and even the tax collector! These contradictions over the decades created confusion and controversy about the dangers of marijuana.

The early "medicinal" uses were not the same as advocates are urging today but included:

- Gastric problems

- Malaria, fever

- Arthritis, general pain or headaches

- Eating disorders

- STDs

- Mental Health

Over the early centuries, hemp developed into one of those standard, "taken for granted" items that many growing industries used or still use where it's legal. Some common but surprising products are textiles; paper, fuel, plastics and some new hemp-food products are in development. Hemp was such a critical crop for a number of purposes (including essential war requirements – rope, etc.) that the government went out of its way to encourage growth. The United States Census of 1850 counted 8,327 hemp "plantations" (minimum 2,000-acre farm) growing cannabis hemp for cloth, canvas and even the cordage used for baling cotton.

The fact that there was a plant for making hemp and one to get a buzz from created quite a bit of confusion when banning it became a political football in the 1920s.

As a cash crop, marijuana growers have had to create special conditions limiting light and dark exposure, and the actual gender of the plant. The female version is the one that is cultivated to take advantage of its psychoactive properties. The plant that once grew wild is now grown in forests shielded by tree top cover, by organized drug cartels and in state-of-the art underground hydroponics labs.

- Cannabis plants produce a unique family of compounds called cannabinoids: cannabidiol (CBD) and delta-9 tetrahydrocannabinol (THC), but only THC is psychoactive. Today, industrial hemp and marijuana are both classified by taxonomists as 'cannabis sativa', a species with hundreds of varieties. Cannabis sativa was once thought to be a member of the mulberry family, but is now considered, along with hops, to belong to the hemp family. Industrial hemp has high CBD and low THC and is bred to maximize fiber, seeds and/ or seed oil, while marijuana varieties seek to minimize CBD and maximize THC (the primary psychoactive ingredient in marijuana).

- While industrial hemp and marijuana may look somewhat alike to an untrained eye, an easily trained eye can easily distinguish the difference.

- The female Cannabis sativa plant not only flowers but also produces hundreds of seeds for further growing. The flowers contain the active THC that produces the end product sold by the dealers for "recreation".

- Industrial cannabis is grown for commercial, non-psychoactive purposes and is where hemp is derived. The level of CBD is high while the THC level is only between 0.05 and 1%.

- Marijuana—from the female plant—called pot, dope, weed or "reefer" has a THC content of 3% to 20% and is the potentially dangerous version of this plant.

- A percentage of the female plants are not pollinated as they grow and are kept apart from the male plants. These infertile plants are the ones that are sold for their active THC content. Others are pollinated to keep the strain going—much like any other crop.

- When prepared properly, the leaves of the female plant also can be converted to hashish—a more powerful form of cannabinoids. Once the male plants are stripped of their pollen they are not viable any longer.

- A *cannabis* plant in the vegetative growth phase of its life requires more than 12–13 hours of light per day to stay vegetative. Flowering usually occurs when darkness equals at least 12 hours per day. The flowering cycle can last anywhere between nine to fifteen weeks, depending on the strain and environmental condition

Marijuana 1930's—1960's: Why Marijuana Became So "Dangerous".

In the years between the early 19th Century and the late 1890's, marijuana was, for a variety of reasons, targeted as dangerous substance "used by minority groups" that made them more than just a threat but liable to become violent after a few puffs. (This is why it acquired the nickname locoweed). The banning began in Utah (Mormons smoked a lot of cannabis) in 1910 and within a decade a dozen more states had banned pot.

By the roaring 20[s] and with Prohibition just around the corner, knowledge of marijuana's $$$$ value (and others like cocaine) flipped it upside down from just a fiber to something more valuable, something illegal that fit the law of supply and demand. The reasons (enjoyment, relaxation) why some cultural groups smoked marijuana were finally obvious and then spread by the time Prohibition was being added to The Constitution. Despite the laws, marijuana "crossed over" permanently in the "roaring 20's" from use by jazz musicians and Hispanic farm workers where it began turning up as a profit center among groups of young white collar and middle class executives.

Marijuana Film Fest

Most Americans (or pot smokers) have seen or heard of an anti-pot film **Reefer Madness** a well-known 1936 propaganda film that shows teenagers who fall into the grip of seedy dope dealers who ply them with pot. The results are suicide, rape, car crashes, and eventually the survivors end up writhing on the floor slowly going insane.

Originally financed by a church group under the title *Tell Your Children*, the message to parents was to teach them about the dangers of cannabis use. The film disappeared for decades, occasionally resurfacing under titles like *Dope Addict, Doped Youth, Love Madness*, and *The Burning Question*. It returned to life as a "comedy" in the 1970s and can be seen on late night cable TV.

Through most of the 20th Century and continuing now, the U.S. government classifies cannabis as a dangerous, addicting, brain-damaging drug. Of all the drugs of abuse that have traveled a very winding road from legal and widespread commercial commodity to the literal source of a drug war, marijuana has the most curious history and causes significant damage both psychologically and neurologically. Why this happens is only being recognized now and how it gets a grip on your brain is explained in depth in **Chapter 2.**

Once the "word" about the psychoactive effect of smoking pot got out, it took less than half a century for marijuana to become the poster child for a good drug gone bad. But unlike the validity given to the apothecaries, marijuana users ignored and flaunted its use in the face of attempts to ban it. The population become skeptical when the authorities make most controversial statements.

Why Does Pot Get You High?

The war on drugs, especially marijuana, that began in the first decade of the 20th century, was largely carried out for political and criminal reasons, but not really justified scientifically until the early 1990's. It was not until then that the psychoactive reaction in the brain to marijuana was revealed and its most active ingredient THC was mapped and understood.

For decades, pot had been considered simply a "loco-weed" by its opponents and a source of pleasure that heightened your senses (i.e. better sex) and helped you mellow out by its advocates. There was no question that something was different about this plant. The search for a new high including smoking everything from banana skins to flowers or just about anything that was rumored to be better (i.e. legal) than pot and not as bad as tobacco.

According to The California Society of Addiction Medicine's Timmen Cermak, M.D.… scientists had always been "curious about how marijuana makes people high. They had known for some time that they were able to isolate a single compound - THC - that produces most of the high…. that comes from the part of the plant that contains an oily resin."

The first important secret that unraveled and led to a theory on why and how marijuana worked appeared appropriately in the 60's. In 1964, just as the pot/LSD, counterculture, hippie, "turn on, tune in, drop out" era was beginning to spread, Rafael Mechoulam, Ph.D. cracked the mystery and revealed the structure of the THC molecule. Dr. Cermak points out "because THC is the primary (but not the only) active ingredient in the cannabis plant, the class of chemicals similar in structure came to be known as cannabinoids or delta-9-tetrahydro*cannabinol* that gave rise to the popular usage as "cannabinoids."

This discovery was a breakthrough that, when studied for several more years concluded: The THC in marijuana alters the brain's activity; and the experience of this changed brain functioning is what people call being "high." What was still unknown was how this process works—for example did the marijuana's cannabinoids travel through the brain looking for preset receptors where other addicting drugs seemed to work?

Not surprising, this was what was happening—sort of. The THC molecules did attach to specific protein molecules dubbed CB1. Think of them as keyholes because only these molecules could fit into the receptors perfectly and then, in effect lock, to keep the brain feeling the effect of the marijuana.

The next question, Dr. Timmen says was obvious. Why were humans outfitted with DNA that led to the construction of bodies and brains that were "hardwired" to attract something whose major use was either to spin into fabric or get people stoned? This puzzled researchers until 1992, when Dr. Mechoulam, the pioneer who had demonstrated the structure of THC, discovered the answer.

We were not built for pot, but rather for another cannabinoid that occurred naturally, and was the same shape for the 'keyhole' receptor cites. In this case Dr. Mechoulam discovered a cannabinoid called 'anandamide' that is built for what we now know is actually a cannabinoid system—a neurotransmitter pathway that is not there for THC, but is used by THC to bring the effect of marijuana into our brains. This is now called the endocannabinoid system.

This is only part of the story of how marijuana does what it does that makes it so attractive to so many people—of all ages. The story, from a more scientific, in-depth point of view, is an important one beyond just marijuana. For example, we now know that the endocannabanoid system has had an important impact on the evolution of insects and humans and everything in between. It is also our largest and most important neurotransmitter system.

Today the questions that these discoveries pose are an integral part of why marijuana is so controversial.

Now That We Know This—Does It Matter?

Today, at least half of all Americans admit to using marijuana once. (It's likely that most did inhale, too.) Marijuana's greatest danger is among adolescents with use at age 13 about 7% but rising to 40% among 17 year olds. Most startling is that in a single day more than 14 million people used pot and about 1/3 did so 20 times or more. It's no surprise that marijuana is a massive addiction and public health issue—especially among adolescents.

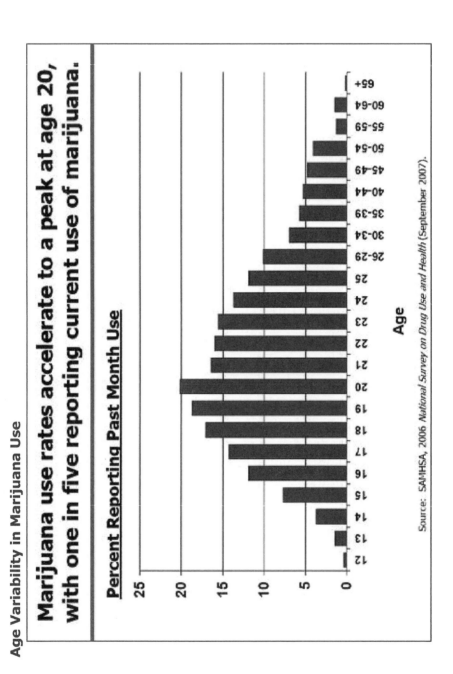

Age Variability in Marijuana Use

Marijuana use rates accelerate to a peak at age 20, with one in five reporting current use of marijuana.

Percent Reporting Past Month Use

Age

Source: SAMHSA, 2006 *National Survey on Drug Use and Health* (September 2007).

Chart From U.S. National Drug Control Policy on number of past marijuana users and other illicit drugs they also use.

Marijuana's banning over the years has not stopped people from trying to make money legitimately with it as a legal drug. It is the number one cash crop in California today grown in the rural areas of Northern California. Taxed to the breaking point, California citizens are seriously considering decriminalizing marijuana.

According to *TIME* Magazine focusing on marijuana's potential to rescue the Golden State's economy,

> *Pot is, after all, California's biggest cash crop, responsible for $14 billion a year in sales, dwarfing the state's second largest agricultural commodity — milk and cream — which brings in $7.3 billion a year, according to the most recent USDA statistics. The state's tax collectors estimate the bill would bring in about $1.3 billion a year in much needed revenue, offsetting some of the billions of dollars in service cuts and spending reductions outlined in the recently approved state budget.*

If there is one thing however that has generated more controversy regarding marijuana is its value as a medical treatment to relieve pain for cancer victims and other uses described below. As a "medicine" it's also quite valuable—In California *"Currently, $200 million in medical-marijuana sales are subject to sales tax."* Despite marijuana's potential as a panacea for financial rescue, pot is basically banned and on the Federal Government's Schedule I drugs reserved for narcotics, opiates and other most dangerous "drugs". Advocates of medical marijuana claim it can cure or treat everything from Alzheimer's to breast cancer and is legally available in 15 states.

The 60's: Dope Is Everywhere

The 1950's and 1960's marked the first time that "pot" began to appear on campuses and among young professionals. It had multiple nicknames, code words or just "dope". What is striking about the next 40 years in the spread of marijuana is that many people felt it was either legal or no more serious than a speeding ticket. Over the next decades pot was used openly and became as ubiquitous as hot dogs and burgers at a barbecue (and was because it caused increased appetite.). Marijuana was and still is a part of the "experience" at rock concerts and is the "joke" in dozens of "stoner" movies made by Cheech and Chong or *Fast Times At Ridgemont High*—that are now cult films on the level of *Reefer Madness*.

One of the other odd aspects of the "new age" where young people held "be-ins" and used drugs to seek a higher consciousness, no one seemed to know where it came from on the street user level. However, at that time networks of marijuana growers and central distribution were starting to grow in South and Central America and states like California that had proper growing climates. Many entrepreneurs, college or young kids with pilot licenses were willing to risk a few years in jail for significant profit. *This was the real beginning when the seemingly benign source of hemp became a very damaging drug.*

Oddly, "maryjane," or whatever it was called was not just illegal in 1960 but had been so for 50 years. Not just "slightly legal" but a full blown narcotic in the same class as heroin, cocaine and synthetic drugs like methamphetamine. Marijuana had been closely regulated for some time and these laws were demanded by the most important law enforcement officials of the time. Still, even today it is widely distributed.

And It Has Succeeded: Marijuana's Legal History

Today the US Drug Enforcement Agency classifies all cannabis sativa varieties as "marijuana." While it is theoretically possible to get permission from the government to grow hemp, DEA would require that fence, razor wire, dogs, guards, and lights secure the field, making it cost-prohibitive.

- Beginning in 1906, the District of Columbia and multiple other states prohibited marijuana. Many of these laws were eventually used to target Mexican workers who crossed the border.

- In 1913, the first laws aimed at preventing "Indian hemp" or any sort of hemp from growing, thus closing that loophole.

- In 1925 United States supported regulation of *Indian hemp*, also known as hashish, in the International Opium Convention. This law prevented hashish from being used.

Uniform State Narcotic Act (1925–1932)

The Uniform State Narcotic Act, first tentative draft in 1925 and fifth final version in 1932, was a result of work by the National Conference of Commissioners on Uniform State Laws. It was argued that the traffic in narcotic drugs should have the same safeguards and the same regulation in all of the states. The committee took into consideration the fact that the federal government had already passed The Harrison Act in 1914 and *The Federal Import and Export Act* in 1922.

The 1936 Geneva Trafficking Convention

In 1936, the Convention for the Suppression of the Illicit Traffic in Dangerous Drugs (1936 Trafficking Convention) was concluded in Geneva. The U.S., led by Harry J. Anslinger, had attempted to include in the treaty the criminalization of all activities – cultivation, production, manufacture and distribution – related to the use of opium, coca (and its derivatives) and cannabis for non-medical and non-scientific purposes. Many countries opposed this and the focus remained on illicit trafficking.

Marijuana Tax Act (1937)

Hemp was grown commercially (with increasing governmental interference) in the United States until the 1950s. The Marijuana Tax Act of 1937, which placed an extremely high tax on marijuana and made it effectively impossible to grow industrial hemp, doomed it. While Congress expressly expected the continued production of industrial hemp, the Federal Bureau of Narcotics lumped industrial hemp with marijuana, as it's successor the US Drug Enforcement Administration, does to this day.

The Marijuana Tax Act of 1937 made possession or transfer of cannabis illegal throughout the United States under federal law, excluding medical and industrial uses, in which an expensive excise tax was required. Annual fees for the tax were $24 ($337 adjusted for inflation) for importers, manufacturers, and cultivators of cannabis, $1 annually ($14 adjusted for inflation) for medical and research purposes, and $3 annually ($42 adjusted for inflation) for industrial uses.

In its 1969 *Leary v. United States* decision, the Supreme Court held the Marijuana Tax Act to be unconstitutional since it violated the Fifth Amendment privilege against self-incrimination. In response, Congress repealed the Marijuana Tax Act and passed the Controlled Substances Act as Title II of the Comprehensive Drug Abuse Prevention and Control Act of 1970, which repealed the Marijuana Tax Act.

Mandatory Sentencing (1952, 1956)

Mandatory sentencing and increased punishment were enacted when the United States Congress passed the Boggs Act of 1952 and the Narcotics Control Act of 1956. The acts made a first time cannabis possession offense a minimum of two to ten years with a fine up to $20,000; however, in 1970, the United States Congress repealed mandatory penalties for cannabis offenses.

Post 1960's

In 1968, the United States Department of the Treasury subsidiary Bureau of Narcotics and the United States Department of Health, Education, and Welfare subsidiary Bureau of Drug Abuse Control merged to create the Bureau of Narcotics and Dangerous Drugs as a United States Department of Justice subsidiary.

In 1973, President Richard Nixon's "Reorganization Plan Number Two" proposed the creation of a single federal agency to enforce federal drug laws and Congress accepted the proposal, as there was concern regarding the growing availability of drugs. As a result, on July 1, 1973, the Bureau of Narcotics and Dangerous Drugs (BNDD) and the Office of Drug Abuse Law Enforcement (ODALE) merged together to create the Drug Enforcement Administration (DEA).

On December 1, 1975 the Supreme Court ruled that it was "not cruel or unusual for Ohio to sentence someone to 20 years for having or selling cannabis."

Mandatory Sentencing and Three-Strikes (1984, 1986)

United States v. Oakland Cannabis Buyers' Cooperative (2001)
In 1996, California voters passed Proposition 215, which legalized medical cannabis. The Oakland Cannabis Buyers' Cooperative,

was created to "provide seriously ill patients with a safe and reliable source of medical cannabis, information and patient support" in accordance with Proposition 215.

Drug Courts

Drug courts are fast growing in number. The first started in 1989; 2140 drug courts were in operation May 2008, with another 284 being planned or developed. They offer offenders charged with less-serious crimes of being under the influence, possession of a controlled substance, or even drug-using offenders charged with a non-drug related crime the option of entering the drug court system in lieu of serving a jail sentence.

Offenders will have to plead guilty to the charge, agree to take part in treatment, regular drug screenings, and regular reporting to the drug court judge for a minimum of one year. Should the offender fail to comply with one or more of the requirements they may be removed from the drug court and incarcerated at the judge's discretion. If they complete the drug court program the charges brought against them are dropped or reduced

Over 30 industrialized democracies do distinguish hemp from marijuana. International treaties regarding marijuana make an exception for industrial hemp.

Marijuana Wars Today:

While the popularly called "drug wars" seem to focus on marijuana, there is no question that it is simply the 800 pound gorilla in the room and it's sitting on cocaine, "legal" prescription medications, over-the counter drugs with alcohol and amphetamine mixtures, and sedatives that are a combination of pain and opioid drugs. There is a drug war taking place globally that involves all these categories of drugs, but marijuana, because it's coming into the U.S. receives most of the headlines.

And of course, there's another reason; the so-called Mexican Drug War is literally an armed civil war between drug "cartels" who grow and import powerful marijuana to many in the US and around the world. At the same time, the Mexican government with American "support" is in a violent, and spreading attack on the cartels but with little success since the US State Department estimates that 70% of illegal drugs grown south of the border end up here. Drug sales may reach as high as $48 billion, much of it in cash that is flown or trucked over the border.

Books, movies, television documentaries have created public awareness of the violence in Mexico and the drug/gang activity in our streets. This makes it all that much harder to recognize that only a few decades ago, smoking a joint at a rock concert was not considered all that serious. The scientific community, especially the addiction specialists were beginning to recognize the potential dangers of cannabis but today, this is no longer "your fathers pot." Today the threats to the health of your family from marijuana are serious.

But this same pattern of "good drugs gone bad" has now spread, especially among adolescents but also to adults and this damage can be just as fatal as a heart attack or a stroke—which they sometimes can cause.

Pills: From The Pharmacy To The Street:

- In 2009, there were 7.0 million (2.8 percent) persons aged 12 or older who used prescription- type psychotherapeutic drugs nonmedically in the past month. These estimates were higher than in 2008 (6.2 million or 2.5 percent), but similar to estimates in 2007 (6.9 million or 2.8 percent).

- Among adolescents aged 12 to 17, the rate of nonmedical use of prescription-type drugs declined from 4.0 percent in 2002 to 2.9 percent in 2008, then held steady at 3.1 percent in 2009

- The young and old appear to have significant risk. Adolescents and elderly, who account for only 13% of the population, receive almost a third of all prescribed medication in the United States, which significantly increases risk for intentional and unintentional misuse.

Earlier we mentioned the influence of the "apothecary" and the role of the pharmacist, who brought a sense of trust and professionalism to the art of compounding drugs or dispensing them accurately. The "malt shop" or drug store with its soda fountain, ice cream and a pharmacy section was central to the lives of teenagers and families for generations. It was hardly linked to drug abuse and addiction, which makes the spread of illicit prescription drug use even more tragic.

Today there are about 269,000 pharmacists, about 2/3 working in retail settings from large markets, retail stores and in small-town drug stores. A pharmacist's education level requires a license and often an advanced degree. Most druggists consider that education and patient counseling is important to promoting safe medication use and is a key aspect of their job. (Establish a relationship with the drug store personnel and don't hesitate to call them with questions.)

While marijuana is still clearly the number one drug of choice other prescription medications, usually pills or liquid, are now approaching marijuana use levels. This pattern of a medication, when taken incorrectly, leading to addiction or overdose is growing. Again, adolescents are a significant part of this group. Anywhere from 8000-10000 adults (over age 12) will use an illicit drug or abuse a prescription drug for the first time. A third who use marijuana for the first time will begin use of prescribed or OTC pain relievers, tranquilizers, stimulants, and sedatives—but not as directed by the doctor or pharmacist.

How have prescription drugs which have been developed to save and rebuild lives, over a few generations, especially the 20th and early 21st centuries, become another source of addiction? This includes pharmaceuticals including painkillers, stimulants, anti-anxiety drugs, weight loss and antidepressants, to name a few categories. (**Section III**)

Ironically the most important reason is simple because prescription drugs, in general "worked" especially in the categories mentioned above. They became an addictive substance as described in **Section II** —because of continued use despite loss of control and disregard for yourself and others.

The main problem with this sort of addiction is that unlike marijuana, prescription drug abuse rests on availability so the user can obtain more. There are two very clear problems here. First the desire for more and more pain killing drugs may be legitimate. Anyone with a severe spinal injury, chronic headaches, or the need to be more focused knows how much certain medication can help. Second your doctor also knows what the proper and legal dose of the medication should be and they have a responsibility to try to treat you with a drug that will not harm you which is why a doctor tries to transition you to an over the counter medication.

If you or someone you care for is teetering on the edge of addiction to pills now is the time to understand the story of how prescription drugs became another chapter in "good drugs gone bad." The drive for the dangerous medication may in the beginning be a legitimate one. In fact, you've discovered that one helps you through the day so obviously a second one can help you through the night. This is common for many of the psychoactive medications that target the central nervous system, and affect the brain as it controls mood, cognitive skills and even your ability to carry out simple tasks or, worse cause an auto accident driving a car while impaired.

It's fairly easy to see how marijuana became a controversial and subsequently an illegal drug. Creating a drug for the "medication" road to a positive solution to a disease requires decades of research and literally "human" trial and error. Because these human trials are targeted toward a correct dose and proper use, often the "street" discovers the misuse. Of course strong warning labels may be required by the FDA but are usually ignored.

Commonly Abused Prescription Medications

Although many prescription medications can be abused, the following three classes are most commonly abused:

Opioids—usually prescribed to treat pain.

CNS depressants—used to treat anxiety and sleep disorders.

Stimulants—prescribed to treat ADHD and narcolepsy.

The Oxycodone Story: A Cautionary and Typical Story

One of the most frequently prescribed and abused painkillers is Oxycodone (a time released version), of the generic version of Oxycontin, which is frequently used for both moderate and severe pain. "Oxy" has a bit of a checkered past. It was developed at the University of Frankfurt (Germany) in 1916 by several scientists, working for the Bayer Co. They decided that one of their main products, **heroin,** was dangerous and addictive (albeit effective). Plan B was to explore the potential of a thebaine, a derivative of opium that seems to have the same analgesic powers but less dependency potential. There is still controversy about this conclusion but ultimately thebain became Oxycodone.

One reason why this conversion was possible is a common trait to all opioids; they change the brain's perception of pain. The drug affects the endogenous opiate system, acting as a thermostat or regulator. Not only has this increased dependency and abuse but also it has created combinations of drugs that have become popular among users. For example, today heroin and cocaine are mixed into a deadly combination called a "speedball". Opioid addiction is also, unfortunately a scenario on several popular television programs that focus on the use of opiates, and the drive for more—but in these cases there is no true damage to these doctors or nurses who seemingly just sail through leaving wreckage in their families or jobs.

It was hoped that a thebaine-derived drug would retain the analgesic effects of morphine and heroin with less dependence. To some extent this was achieved, as the synthetic oxycodone did have the same immediate effect as heroin or morphine and it did not last as long. While Oxycontin was first sold in Europe in the late 1910, it was not available in the US until 1939. It quickly climbed the abused drug bestseller list. The International Narcotics Control Board estimates that at least 11 tons of oxycodone were produced worldwide in 1998, but in the next decade the yearly "yield" was more than 75.2 tons in 2007 and also the largest consumption per capita. The pharmaceutical manufacturers recognized that they had a hot drug on their hands but also a dangerous one. For example in 2001, Purdue Pharma discontinued the 160 mg. strength because of the "possibility of illicit use of tablets of such high strength." The Drug Enforcement Agency (DEA) denied that it had made this request—implying that Purdue knew it was a dangerous drug.

Given its roots and its wide use, it's not surprising to know that not only is Oxycontin the best selling brand name painkiller in the US but also its revenues were above $2.5 billion. Over the last decade as Oxy was used more and more and in combination with drugs like acetaminophen (Tylenol), making it a quick way to get high and more importantly, wealthy. A recent arrest in Rhode Island netted 4200 Oxycontin pills said to be worth at least $250,000 on the street.

Above is a typical story of hundreds of drugs produced for the benefit of the greatest number of people—that takes a sharp turn and goes off the tracks, putting it into the same category of marijuana. It is a drug that is now both used for legitimate and illegal purposes.

On one hand this class of narcotic pain killers and combo drugs have salvaged millions of lives that might have kept them from work or a normal life. Yet, the biological hook up for a drug like Oxycontin, or sedatives, anti-anxiety and mental health medications is pretty well understood and it has created an imbalance in the supply and demand side of unintended drug dependency and addiction.

As a result, there are three primary methods that patients use to obtain this and similar drugs when doctors limit its use.

These Include:

- Number one on this list is widely known to physicians and pharmacists—**doctor shopping.** Most patients quickly figure out that MDs are busy and if they know medical jargon they are likely to get them a new prescription. Unfortunately, the patients are talking to a doctor who has never met them and this continues in a circle until they burn out.

- Second is *weekend* **MD shopping** when most doctors are off and a resident unfamiliar with the case gets a phone request from a pharmacy or the patient for a refill. Fortunately many doctors and hospitals have a policy prohibiting narcotic medicine on the weekends or someone familiar with the case is contacted. The patients are told to go to the ER. Doctor shopping also occurs at all times but is a bit more difficult since the patient's primary physician is available and few doctors will write prescriptions for someone elses patient.

- Third and most disturbing source of illegal prescription drugs is through the **Internet.** No one really knows how many online outlets for medications exist. Getting a prescription is relatively easy, since patients have all sorts of excuses from cost to the classic "my dog ate my tranquilizers." Actually, pills sold on the Internet often are either counterfeit or simply weaker or "look-alike" versions of the real thing.

The use of prescription medication has continued to grow with 2.3 billion prescriptions dispensed in 2008. Most visits to the doctor (74%) ended with a script being handed over. Painkillers, followed by cholesterol control and antidepressant drugs were the leading category. In other words 2 of 3 had abuse potential.

Hospital outpatient visits resulted in 280 million prescriptions written except in this case the painkillers were at the top of the list followed by antidepressants and then lipid lowering drugs.

In Section II of this book other prescription medications are fully described. Medications such as pain killers, sedatives, antidepressants, stimulants and tranquilizers have likely saved and turned around more lives than harmed by misuse. Even if you are told that it takes time for a drug and your body to connect properly, let your doctor know if you are having problems or if you suspect you are becoming dependent on the drug. Read the package information and make sure you understand it.

Over The Counter: From Drug Store Shelves To Schoolyards

- 40 percent of teens feel that OTC medicines are much safer than illegal drugs

- 31 percent of teens agree that using OTC and Rx medications is okay "once in a while"

- 55 percent of teens do not strongly feel that it is risky to use cough medicine to get high

- 10 percent of teen's reports that they use cough medicine to get high

An attorney, who works with teenagers who have been abused, told the author that his "clients are frequently in trouble but do not use the drugs that you might suspect—heroin, or cocaine." Those drugs are considered "old school" by today's kids regardless of gender or ethnic background, and also are expensive from their point of view. The teenagers today shop for their buzz in Wal-Mart, Walgreens, or large supermarket chains. This is one of the worst examples of commonly used drugs morphing into a drug of abuse—that many parents only find out when they read an article in a parenting magazine or at a PTA meeting.

For boomers, this may seem to be an odd choice of drugs to abuse since cough syrup and other OTCs were traditionally the purview of the local "winos" or the black sheep uncle who was drunk and continually nodded off, pitching forward into the pumpkin pie at Thanksgiving. It was good for a laugh but not taken too seriously.

Unfortunately, the spread of over-the counter medications is growing each year for one reason: availability. In a recent study, 56% of teenagers, who are the majority of OTC users preferred them to illegal drugs simply because they are easy to obtain. Others mentioned both the Internet and their family's medicine closet as a source.

Because prescription medications can be expensive and hard to get, those who continue to search for a high have found an entire new, largely unregulated and seemingly endless source of drugs. These are now the hottest places to shop for legal uppers and downers. Generally, teens don't recognize that OTC meds are very dangerous when dosages or other drugs are mixed—after all they are given spoonfuls of these drugs as kids and their (trusted) parents dispensed them.

The most dangerous OTC medication is anything that has a chemical called **Dextromethorphan (DXM),** which is found in more than 100 non-prescription cough and cold medications. DXM is the active ingredient found in OTC cough and cold medications. When taken in recommended doses, these medications are safe and effective.

These include:

- Robitussin

- Nyquil

- Vicks

- Formula 44

- Coricidin HBP Cough and Cold tablets

The list of abused OTCs goes far beyond DXM including sleep aids, weight loss, energy boosters (a very new craze), athletic anti-pain creams, diet pills, sleep aids, and motion sickness medication. According to treatment counselors and doctors adolescents who take large doses of sea sickness meds can experience hallucinations. Sleep aids are especially dangerous since they can lead to an overall weakness in the body and even a serious condition called narcolepsy—sudden bouts of falling asleep—for example while driving.
Anyone with a teenager recognizes that often they are speaking a different language than you are (with certain exceptions that include requests) and computer-speak has added to your illiteracy. In this case,

it's a good idea to learn the nicknames (and code) that adolescents have for o-t-c drugs. The most important drug that should raise a red flag in your direction is anything that has to do with DXM.

Most common nicknames include:

- Skittles
- Triple C's
- Vitamin D
- Tussin

Parents have a strong challenge where OTCs are concerned. Not only are they inexpensive, come in handy pill forms and best of all for an adolescent in most cases, they are legal. The DEA simply "keeps watch on them as a drug of concern" and DXM remains widely available. Some pharmacies are keeping any drugs with DXM behind the pharmacy counters but this has a minimal effect. Literally, any adolescent can buy a bottle and go on the Internet for "recipes".

Recently community and big box pharmacies, at the request of local police have begun to keep the DXM bottles or liquid behind the counter but other combination drugs are generally available on the open shelves.

DXM can be a killer, depending on the amount taken. Essentially DXM is a brain busting medication and its effect can be compared to PCP or the animal tranquilizer, ketamine. Everything from inability to walk, talk numbness, gastrointestinal effects and heart and blood pressure effects can occur. Combined with other drugs such as decongestants it can cause brain death.

More To Come:

Trends and statistics are found in more depth in Appendix A, for both adolescents and adults, however the message of this chapter is to demonstrate just how easy it is for a very useful and legal drug to become abused and lead to a great deal of addiction. There are several more drugs of abuse that will be discussed in greater depth in section two of this book and followed by the UF Addiction Recovery program.

Other drugs that are well known to be abused by people of all ages and genders are addictive and also "underestimated" and discussed in Section Two. They include:

- Tobacco

- Alcohol

- Binge Drinking

- Club Drugs (Ecstasy-MDMA)

- Steroids

- Inhalants

- NSAIDS

- Heroin

- Opioids

- Methamphetamine

- PCP

- LSD

- Hallucinogens

Chapter Five: Drugs and The Family

Part One:
Worrying About Your
Children and Addiction

What Should You Consider?

If you suspect your child or adolescent is taking drugs, using alcohol or even popping pills, you are probably too late to begin a home *prevention* program but not too late to have an *intervention*. You will know very quickly when you confront them with your suspicions and/or evidence which choice to make. If their reaction is similar to their general behavior (i.e. mumbling or grunting something vague like "right"), you may have less to worry about. As a parent you recognize this as actually a *normal* teen response to virtually everything from being told to clean their room, do homework or take out the trash. Teens often seem to be orbiting Saturn when talking to a parent— you were a teen once and know what's normal or not.

However you *may* have a problem if they react strongly, responding with anger, defensiveness and door slamming as they retreat to their room, usually tossing something to illustrate their shock that you would even think something this outrageous.

To be fair, they may just be angry (or they may be high at the time and have tuned you out in favor of The Simpsons). Depending on the age of your child, and if you suspect drug use, prepare yourself for a sort of guerrilla war full of skirmishes, ceasefires and personal worry—and a significant amount of amateur advice from friends and family members.

Why Do People *Start* Taking Drugs?

Before you launch a battle with your teen over possible drinking or drug use, it's important to arm yourself with some basic information and possible strategies to keep yourself on an effective path. We have answers about what various drugs do to our brains and why they create a drive for more drugs despite knowing that it can and will cause harm. We closely track who is using which drug for public education campaigns. *We know how alcohol, marijuana, cocaine, stimulants, sedative, opioids, prescription drugs and the OTCs that line the pharmacy shelves affect us, but we are not exactly sure why people start for the first time. Is it curiosity, social pressure, lack of judgment?*

Why does one person stop taking narcotic pain meds when their injury is healed but another does not? Are some people predisposed to marijuana, but not opioids? Is there a "drug abuser gene" just waiting to be turned on? Even when we have very hard data that is repeated in study after study, the conclusions we draw are more "likely" to be true than definitive. There are two basic answers—especially for adolescents.

Yearly studies conducted by NIDA, CDC and other agencies seek to find out first what the *perceived availability* of a drug is to different age groups.

They ask "How difficult do you think it would be for you to get each of the following types of drugs, if you wanted some?"

The answer categories are "probably impossible," "very difficult," "fairly difficult," "fairly easy," and "very easy." For 8th and 10th graders, an additional answer category—"can't say, drug unfamiliar"—is offered and included in the calculations.

So, one important reason people and teens start taking a drug is obvious (on one level). It's there!

This reason—perceived availability, also enables someone with a genetic predisposition to take the leap off the edge of the cliff despite some warning.

For example: Statistically, we know that children of alcoholics are more likely to follow their parents on that route. In fact, according to the American Academy of Child and Adolescent Psychiatry, one in five Americans lived with an alcoholic while growing up and "alcoholism runs in families, and children of alcoholics are four times more likely than other children to become alcoholics. Most children of alcoholics have experienced some form of neglect or abuse."

Why then, would someone drink, with those odds, knowing what life in that environment could be? Having genetic predispositions, specific to alcohol, why do people begin the abuse of other drugs?

Studies and years of clinical treatment have suggested a common thread—how one is "initiated" into the process. What are the circumstances that led to that first joint or the first pill? *It may be social, or a result of peer pressure or simply something to try because "everyone else is doing it."*

A second, stronger factor that could entice an adolescent into a first drug or alcohol use is *perceived risk.* The rule of thumb is, as perceived risk goes up, use of a drug goes down. Of course this could be reversed—use goes up with lowered risk fear, but education and honesty about drug use is more likely to have a positive effect. Consider the anti-smoking campaigns or litter reduction programs that have been so successful.

To prevent use of drugs, it's very important to dispel myths and to put it honestly—**don't lie**, especially because prevention of initiation is much more successful than cessation. Point out that propaganda like the *Reefer Madness* film and other over-the-top, skewed information is untrue and supply factual information that is easily available from The National Institute of Drug Abuse (NIDA).

One approach is a method that is becoming more reliable: look at what we think makes people drug abusers—as a group. What do they have in common or what is their trigger that led them into drugs of addiction? This approach has been employed to study aging populations. For example, the longest lived populations are female Japanese, whose life style and diet is particularly healthy and Americans, who have more people living to 100 years old.

This tells us something about the epidemiology or demographics of these groups, but not everything. There are many people who do not 'live long and prosper' in these countries.

In relating this to drug use among adolescent and adults, there are four specific characteristics that almost always are present in the life of a drug abuser or someone who progresses to addiction for you to keep in mind.

1. *Environment*: What was the house and family like growing up? Was there an alcoholic, a step-parent? Words count—was home-life like a war? What was the neighborhood like? Who were your peers and what did you do—this is a major factor.

2. *Genetic or Biological*: Genetic pre-disposition increases vulnerability to the disease of addiction or reaction to a drug.

3. *Sociocultural* (i.e. Americans always want more things faster and more fun)

4. *Psychological*: Our temperaments are different and so are our reactions to drugs; we are all wired differently due to our past—perhaps abused as kids or overindulged.

How Do You Prevent Drug Addiction?

As mentioned above, preventing initiation into drugs–especially after the fact is very difficult. However, locking the door when you've gone over the edge with a child, will always lead to a more complicated problem to solve that can break up families, cause divorces, and even see your child in Juvee hall (juvenile detention).

Below are a few questions for you to consider and also some general ideas to help with young people at any stage. Keep these "stages of vigilance" in mind, too:

- **Primary Prevention:** Just as you would stop any disease, the same goes for drugs. Reduce any possible exposure that you can.

- **Secondary Prevention:** High risk adolescents and even younger children who may have genetic predispositions should be identified and prevention work started with the child.

- **Tertiary Prevention:** A child at this level who is discovered or found to be using drugs, must get treatment at some level. Parents have to be vigilant and ready to act quickly. Watch out for your own denial.

One of the challenges parents face is when the "drug problem" may or may not be present. No one lives in a one-size-fits-all solution. Read each and see whether or not you agree and how you might handle the situation:

1. Is It OK To Search?

Would you go through your child's drawers, closets, clothing, book bag and car if you were suspicious? Would you do this if you thought your son or daughter was hanging out with a druggie group? Or not—just to make you feel better, perhaps because of a drug related incident with a friend's child? Add to that, even though you are suspicious, their *behavior hasn't changed*; they are still on the honor roll and play field hockey. What do you think?

Search: Yes   No
Don't Search?   Yes   No

Recommendation: Yes—search. Unequivocally. Explain that it is your house and you reserve the right to determine what is in the house. Explain it in a kind, loving way. No locks are on the door—but be polite—knock and wait. Don't be a SWAT Team.

2. When Is It Time To Have "The Talk" And Which One?

If you are a parent "the talk" is never fun on any topic from sex, money, a drivers license, restrictions to friends, or attending vague social events (i.e. sleepovers) alone. Each talk is inevitable. Unfortunately, a teenager knows that they have the ultimate card to play and use it: "You did it, too," they reply as an answer to anything. Now you have to make a decision. Do you simply say what your parents likely said: "Because I'm your mother/father and I say so!" How's that working out for you? With today's adolescents, probably not too well.

Let's be honest, they will have a good answer for anything you say, and usually based on information that is right at their thumbs, using their smart-phones or in their room with the PC when you are asleep. They can even tweet their friends in the middle of your conversation to get back-up advice without you knowing.

Further, the truth may be that you do drink wine at the table or have a cocktail after work. Just looking at pictures of yourself in the 60's or 70's might suggest to the sophisticated kids of today that if you looked like *that* you must have been stoned.

The first choice—pulling rank—usually has some short-term success since you can take away the car keys, computer or cell phone and simply avoid more confrontation and arguing. After all, things like this have usually calmed down in a few days. That, however, might be in the past.

Perhaps your teen's circumstances have changed and even though your child looks the same to you, they may be running with a new group of people. How do you know she's not going to school and changing clothes, skipping class after checking in at home room? Should you have the "talk" immediately or just try to survive until they leave for college? And which talk is more important— sex or drugs?

When Do You Have The Sex & Drugs Talk?

Age 10
Age 13

Recommendation: Unfortunately you must have it earlier than you want to. Start at ten years old, but no later than middle school. Kids listen even when you think they aren't listening. Keep the three level approaches above in mind. Talk about more than the "heavy stuff". For example, after school activities or teachers they like or don't. Don't lie because they know it and that hurts your credibility.

There are dozens of books, organizations and rehabilitation centers that are full of advice and treatment to combat the spreading use of illegal drugs—especially those created by adolescents from over the counter cough syrups with DXM. The main problem with most "five ways to tell if an adolescent is stoned" anti-drug material is that the advice falls into several, simple either/or categories that may not help satisfy your fears or give you interactive tools to use with your child. Additionally the questions you may need to answer are usually related to where your child is developmentally, including age and level of social maturity or judgment.

Problems you may encounter as a result of any type of drug use in the home (parents too!) require solutions that fit the circumstances within the family. Is the family intact or is it a single parent family? What are the economic circumstances in the home? How much supervision does your child have?

3: Which Drug Threatens Your Family Most?

Because this is a common question many people think the answer is obvious; marijuana or tobacco, after all they seem to get the most media time. You are wrong—think about this for a moment. Which substance of abuse is most likely to be a part of your family life and somewhat easy for your child to obtain? This drug's use is everywhere and the fallout from its abuse can lead to death, violence and crime for "users".

The answer is **alcohol** *and is by far the most dangerous drug for your kids and you.* And it also can be the one drug that your kids are seriously abusing right under your nose. (When confronted you can also count on your child to use the "you do it card" here, too.) How likely is your child to become involved in underage alcohol use— here are just a few stats to help you measure the odds:

According to the **Centers for Disease Control** (CDC) "alcohol is the most commonly used and abused drug among youth in the United States, more than tobacco and illicit drugs."

• Although drinking by persons under the age of 21 is illegal, people aged 12 to 20 years drink 11% of all alcohol consumed in the United States.

• More than 90% of this alcohol is consumed in the form of binge drinking.

• On average, underage drinkers consume more drinks per drinking occasion than adult drinkers.

• In 2008, there were approximately 190,000 emergency rooms visits by persons under age 21 for injuries and other conditions linked to alcohol.

• The **2009 Youth Risk Behavior Survey** found that among high school students, during the past 30 days:

• 42% drank some amount of alcohol.

• 10% drove after drinking alcohol.

• 28% rode with a driver who had been drinking alcohol.

In 2009, the **Monitoring The Future Survey** reported that 37% of 8th graders and 72% of 12th graders had tried alcohol, and 15% of 8th graders and 44% of 12th graders drank during the past month.

What Do All These Numbers Mean?

Just like kids are attracted by perceived availability, they are also attracted to a drug by its *perceived risk*. This is critical and also explains why, as you'll see below, the numbers of adolescents who abuse drugs varies widely, drug by drug. This is how their attitude is measured. When discussing drugs with your children deal with specific drugs, a more concrete approach.

The numbers reflect a few things; most drugs of abuse appear on the scene and after a sort of "grace period" appear on the radar as dangerous substances. If an adolescent has toyed with drug use, the past is the best predictor of the future, and will likely try again until caught. Most dangerously, a child's brain is not fully developed and exposure to drugs or other toxins can be permanently damaging.

In light of these overwhelming and frightening facts and that your kids may have seen you drink frequently, this is a very different situation than any other drug use. Alcohol is everywhere and you may have given them some wine or a little champagne at a party or wedding. You've sent a message that in small doses this is not dangerous. What should you do?

Do not go extreme: Don't lock the liquor cabinet, measure the alcohol in the house, pre-inspect their friend's homes, or breathalyze all boyfriends before and after each date.

Do not overdo the message you send: When it comes to drinking and driving you want them to tell us the truth— different impression—don't invent an image.

Remain calm: Try to keep the conversation focused on your child, the illegality of alcohol and consequences.

4. Why/When Should You Have Concerns?

Two different aspects of this question should be considered carefully. First, there is the common list of statistics (above) that is designed to scare any parent. The consequences of underage drinking can and do potentially lead to horrific consequences. The CDC lists just a few that you may decide are enough to keep a tight rein on your child. While the stats are daunting, they are not reason enough to add more door locks. Still, these are clichés but may have an element of truth:

- School problems, such as higher absences and poor or failing grades.

- Social problems, such as fighting and lack of participation in youth activities.

- Legal problems, such as arrest for driving or physically hurting someone while drunk.

- Physical problems, such as hangovers or illnesses.

- In 2009, 46% of high school students had sexual intercourse and 13.8% had four or more sex partners during their life. Prior to the sexual activity, 21.6% drank alcohol or used drugs. Only 38.9% used a condom.

- Physical and sexual assault.

- Higher risk for suicide and homicide.

- Alcohol-related car crashes and other unintentional injuries, such as burns, falls, and drowning.

- Memory problems.

- Abuse of other drugs.

- Changes in brain development that may have life-long effects.

- Death from alcohol poisoning.

- In general, the risk of youth experiencing these problems is greater for those who binge drink than for those who do not binge drink.

- Youth who start drinking before age 15 years are five times more likely to develop alcohol dependence or abuse later in life than those who begin drinking at or after age 21 years.

There are two problems with these lists. First, they are overkill. If your child or teenager is injured, sick or changing in ways suggested, it is likely that something else besides alcohol or drug use is provoking their behavior and that they may need professional help. Second, when read as a whole, this type of statistics can provoke overreaction on your part leading to alienation or pushing kids into a period of risky experimentation.

In shaping your response, consider the factor that normal teenagers (whom we know from personal experience) are convinced that they are indestructible and safe from risk.

What is the practical and effective method of coping, especially if you have some actual evidence of alcohol or drug use?

Recommendation: AVOID putting them in a position of lying (depending the severity of the evidence). You must be ready to act if they are deceitful, but on the other hand they also should feel they can call you for help.

Part Two:
Avoiding a Drug or Alcohol Disaster

Worrying (Realistically) About Your Children and Addiction:

The Q&A's in Part One are not designed to scare you or to turn you into some sort of tough-love, boot-camp drill sergeant. Instead, it's important to bring some reality about preventing a disaster into your life and avoid tragedy. It's critical to begin and continue thinking about this subject rationally, especially if you are a baby boomer whose slogan was "sex, drugs and rock & roll" or a Gen Xer who is now an overscheduled soccer mom or a dual profession parent who fears they aren't giving enough quality time to their kids.

It's not likely that you will find yourself in some of the situations where the exercises in Part One are possibly accurate and you agree with them. However, if something does happen and your child is harmed by driving drunk or injures someone else, the fallout will be catastrophic—so considering these worst cases is a smart idea—be ahead of the curve.

Behind Door # 2: More Danger:

While above we discuss alcohol's wide use, the most abused substance—the one that affects teens and should have you worrying just as much—is the misuse of over the counter drugs and prescription medication. These are in some ways, parent proof. Unlike tobacco or marijuana use, every time your child or a friend goes to the drug store they can walk out with something that gets them high and the symptoms are not simple to detect.

In chapter four, you found information on how drugs such as prescription stimulants used for ADHD and, of course, marijuana became so widely used and those numbers are growing, too. This disturbing trend, especially non-medical use of opioid prescription drugs (painkillers like oxycodone) has risen and will continue because they are easier to obtain. Further, these drugs and the ones made from OTCs, are growing in both use and danger because the recipes can be found on the Internet and they are not just street drugs anymore, but everywhere. A vast majority of adolescents (56%) feel

OTCs are easier to get than street drugs and 40% feel they are safer than illegal drugs. Additionally, 10 percent of teens report that they use cough medicine to get high.

Teens today also use inhalants—household products such glue, nail polish remover and cleaning solvents—along with "club drugs" like Ecstacy (MDMA) that are fully described later.

Talk The Talk:

Above we emphasize the importance of talking to your kids and suggest some methods. The abuse of alcohol and OTCs is the best place to begin the talk about drugs for at least one reason— you probably know more about these two subjects than the others. Today's marijuana is not remotely the same strength or from a point of origin that you might have smoked in the dorm while listening to Iron Butterfly play "Ina Gadda Vida" ceaselessly. Today's marijuana is grown by sophisticated, experienced pot farmers all over the world and in hybrid forms, just the way an agribusiness company alters the sweetness of corn or the color of tomatoes. You are not alone and the "drug scene" has changed to a virtual war, so don't try to "walk the walk", your kids will know.

According to Teen Help (www.teenhelp.com),

> *One of the biggest problems with curbing teen OTC drug use is the fact that so few teens know about the dangers. Drug education programs focus mainly on illegal drugs and, likewise, parents tend to focus mainly on the dangers of illegal drugs like marijuana (which is also increasing in popularity among teens).*

While the vast majority of parents do report speaking to their children about the dangers of marijuana, not many talk about OTCs. The reason is simple, it's likely that mom or dad can talk with experience about alcohol on some level, but the reality is that OTC info is a mystery.

Here are some talking points that you can use to start the talk or at least have background facts like above to "talk the talk" credibly:

How and where these are sold?

This is relatively simple. Internet searching through key words like **over the counter drug abuse** or **teen drug abuse** is easy and can get you some general material. The best resource in any town is likely only a few moments away. Your local pharmacist—at a large or small store—knows what is going on and if you call ahead and discuss your apprehension, he/she will be happy to talk with you in most cases. Major organizations, like the American Academy of Child and Adolescent Psychiatry (http://www.aacap.org/), have web sites with excellent information for parents to use in a talk.

Initiating the talk:

There are two ways to start a talk on drug abuse. The first is to seize the opportunity that a "teachable moment" might provide. This might unfortunately include an overdose by a classmate, an arrest of another teen for selling drugs, or an automobile accident involving drinking and causing severe injury or death or even a friend who is "in trouble—pregnant."

A good place to start may make you cringe because there might be an echo in your brain that reminds you of the "talk" you received as a teen from your parents. Was it a simple "OK" let's sit down and I'm going to deliver a lecture on sex-which may really have been more like "here's what every boy wants" and then says to you, "now ask any question you want". And there it was, the talk is over, about 25% went into your brain. The problem is that the rest came from your friends.

The absolute best way to have a useful and effective talk about drugs (and sex) is when a teachable moment occurs, especially if you are prepared. A good opportunity for a teachable moment is when it is unplanned. For example, driving by an accident and commenting about safety measures, drunk driving or some other fact you've read. You are likely to get an eye-roll, but at least you've opened a door for more talk later.

Other moments include:

- Watching TV or a movie—especially the typical teen movie today, with alcohol and drug use. Don't censor—use this teachable moment.

- Before a big event like the prom.

- Intervene early.

- Pick up on something that they may be studying in school—biology or science.

- Try to have a "how was your day" talk at home.

- Celebrities seem to go to rehab stints frequently, but come out heroes (unless they are rock stars and die first). Seize on the difference between a young celeb that seems to be in trouble all of the time and someone else who is talented, successful and is only in the headlines for something positive.

- If a celebrity gets out of rehab and then gets back on the team or makes new TV shows, the message to a teen is that maybe it's all right to abuse substances. It's important to point out the better role model.

OK-YOU'VE WALKED THE WALK:

It's certainly unrealistic to think that all of the above can be accomplished in a day, week, month or year. You have to begin prevention of drug abuse while children are small, just as they would be treated by a primary pediatrician; certain information during primary years, secondary and tertiary. The goal is to reduce the chance of allowing a child to become high risk.

Just like there are rules for virtually any aspect of life, it's important to establish them where drugs and medication are concerned:

- Set rules around the home.

- Having a consequence and sticking to it.

- The message is in how you live—what is your attitude toward medicine?

- Talking to your MD.

- When are they at risk?

- Defining one child from another-physical and emotional factors.

- If it's in Walgreens, is it safe?

- Can my wife or I create family risk if we use medication and alcohol frequently?

- Are we setting up a subtle (positive) attitude towards drugs that we all might share?

- Can we give Jimmy the cough syrup we got Suzie who is a different age?

- Obvious safety steps but special measures to take (anaphylactic shock).

- Medications and Traveling.

- Precautions.

- Emergencies.

Here is information anyone should be aware of from current data in the 2010 - Monitoring The Future Survey. The complete data is in Appendix A.

Marijuana use, which had been rising among teens for the past two years, continued to rise in 2010 in all prevalence periods for all three grades. This stands in stark contrast to the long, gradual decline that had been occurring over the preceding decade.

Of relevance, perceived risk for marijuana has been falling in recent years. Of particular relevance, *daily marijuana use* increased significantly in all three grades in 2010; and stands at 1.2%, 3.3%, and 6.1% in grades 8, 10, and 12.

In other words, nearly one in sixteen high school seniors today is a current daily, or near-daily, marijuana user.

After a decline of several years in perceived risk for *ecstasy*, which we had been warning could presage a rebound in use, its use does now appear to be rebounding.

Alcohol use, including *binge drinking,* continued its longer term decline among teens, reaching historically low levels in 2010. Use has been in a long-term pattern of decline since about 1980, with the interruption of a few years in the early 1990s in which alcohol use increased along with the use of cigarettes and almost all illicit drugs.

Among 12th graders in 1980, 41% admitted to having five or more drinks in a row on at least one occasion in the two weeks prior to the survey (what we call binge drinking). This statistic fell to 28% by 1992, prior to the rebound in the 1990s, but has now fallen further reaching 23% in 2010—a marked improvement.

After decelerating considerably in recent years, the long-term decline in *cigarette* use, which began in the mid-1990s, came to a halt in the lower grades in 2010. Indeed, both 8th and 10th graders showed evidence of an increase in smoking in 2010, though the increases did not reach statistical significance. Perceived risk and subsequently disapproval had both leveled off some years ago.

Because marijuana is by far the most prevalent drug included in the *any illicit drug* use index, an increase in prevalence occurred for that index as well as for marijuana. The proportions using *any illicit drug other than marijuana* had been declining gradually since about 2001, but no further decline occurred in 2010.

There was a significant increase in *heroin use using a needle* among 12th graders in 2010, with annual prevalence rising from 0.3% in 2009 to 0.7% in 2010. However, because there was no simultaneous change in use in the lower grades nor any change in attitudes or beliefs that might explain such a change, we believe there is a good possibility that the change is due to chance sample fluctuation.

Cocaine and *powder cocaine* use continued gradual declines in all 12th graders in 2010, with annual prevalence falling from 9.7% in 2009 to 8.0% in 2010.

What About Home Drug Testing? Should Parents Consider It?

Professionally administered drug testing is a part of our culture now. For example workplace drug testing is so common that most people simply consider it a part of holding down a job today. In fact, many, many companies post signs indicating that they have a "drug-free workplace" as a positive promotion to customers.

But, what about home drug testing? The "home testing" industry has also grown in multiple areas over the past few decades. Pregnancy tests compete with each other and home DNA kits are a growth industry—for $80 you can determine paternity of a child and genetic risk testing for the home is on the horizon.

Home drug testing to combat drug abuse, however, has become controversial and a hot button among addiction specialists who are asked about this frequently. One reason the question comes up is that some communities have actually set up programs that provide kits for parents at no cost. The police department in a Long Island, NY town gave away 16,000 kits that used litmus paper and a thermometer to test urine for six different drugs including methamphetamine, marijuana, heroin, Vicodin and Xanax. Since the program started they claim parents have "picked up" nearly 450 positive readings.

When the author is asked this question, or if he approves of home drug testing he offers several things for the parent consider:

1   Why does the parent feel a need to do this? Do they have a "suspicion or actual evidence of drug or alcohol use?"
2   Do they know anything about the physical or emotional signs of drug abuse?
3   Do they know how to cheat on these kits—they can bet if their kid is using they know how to beat the test.
4   These tests—like pregnancy tests—are not 100% accurate and can show false positives. What will you do and how will you feel if you accuse your child and they are innocent?
5   They don't cover all drugs. Kids know which ones and will stay away from those.
6   Think twice about the message you are sending your child. It's a flashpoint issue and the dangers of making a mistake can fracture the family.

Home drug testing is not a good idea and even among Board Certified experts in Addiction Medicine there is further training required to be certified to interpret drug testing! Also, there is very little scientific data that it curbs drug abuse. It is the job of a qualified medical professional to administer and interpret and should only be done if your child is clearly in trouble. If you are so concerned that you are considering disrupting your home then you are concerned enough to call your doctor.

Section II:
A Guide to the Most Abused,
or Dangerous Drugs

In the previous chapters of this book, our goal has been to provide parents and their families with an in-depth examination of today's growing—and quite common—use and abuse of both illicit and "legal" drugs. Our second objective has been to accomplish this goal in a straightforward method and tone. Unfortunately increased drug abuse, according to research studies, government surveys, and criminal involvement does not seem to be slowing down and we at University of Florida's Florida Recovery Center (FRC) are treating more adults and adolescents each year.

Frequently we treat drug users who are addicted to one or more drugs that range from multiple varieties of prescription medication to take them up or down, cough syrup to "robo-trip" on, over the counter drugs called "Skittles," inhalants mixed with paint thinner for a powerful high, LSD to take on an hallucinogenic trip, today's souped-up and brand-name marijuana, and of course, the leaders in the personal damage categories, alcohol, steroids and/or tobacco.

Other information in earlier chapters prior to this section, including a short history of drug abuse and an introduction to the scientific aspects of addiction will help you answer questions when you are talking to a child or having "the talk." The inclusion of some material in more than one place has been done purposely to let the reader "dip in" for quick reference or read the narrative.

What follows is a reference guide to the most commonly abused drugs and medications however; it is not simply a list. We have organized this section in two ways.

- Some medications are essentially the same when it comes to their effects because they are in a common "class". For example, several medications cause sedation and another highly addictive group is strong painkillers based on a biological effect. They are each profiled as a group.

- Major drugs of abuse like cocaine, marijuana and some rarely profiled drugs like Khat (herbs) are individually described.

Alcohol

Quick Facts: Alcohol is the most abused substance on the planet and it has been in the lead for longer than most think. In **Section I,** there are facts and a narrative that also focuses on alcohol use in the United States. The following "quick facts" that cover the "Ancient Period" will give you a little more historical context to the continued popularity of drinks that contain alcohol.

- **Egypt**: It is believed that the Egyptians were considered the first civilization to home-brew alcohol in large quantities and use it in most of their religious ceremonies, especially one for Osiris, "the God of Beer".

- **China**: Evidence exists that as early as 7000 BC, China was the first society to ferment rice, honey, and fruit to create an alcoholic drink.

- **India:** India also was an early brewer—perhaps from 3000 BC - 2000 BC creating "sura", a mixture of rice meal, wheat, sugar cane, grapes & other fruits.

- **Babylon**: The Babylonians (2700 BC) were also very fond of beer, but made sure they were covered by producing wine and adding wine gods and goddesses to their list of deities.

- **Greece**: Always a leader in pleasurable activities, the Greeks by 1700 BC had turned wine into an industry and wine was used at every possible opportunity; as medicine, with meals, and of course, religious events.

- **Rome**: Bacchus, the god of wine, had a cult following and was also known to the Greeks as Dionysus. His main function was to enable the population to "free one's normal self by madness, ecstasy, or wine."

Where It Comes From: Alcohol is not only toxic by itself in high doses but at low doses can be toxic if taken with pain medications, sleeping pills and even OTC medicine like Benadryl. The perceived effect is to relax the drinker, but its chemical composition actually is doing more to the drinker's brain and body. The main ingredient is "ethyl alcohol" and is produced by the fermentation of yeast, sugars and starches. Ethyl alcohol is a close cousin to ethanol (used for fuel) and creates this intoxicating effect found in beer, wine, and liquor.

Sometimes called "liquid courage", when alcohol is used short-term it can reduce anxiety by effecting small changes in the brain, but long-term use can provoke anxiety and panic. Alcohol is good in the moment, but is also very insidious. For example, a small amount of alcohol will leave the body about a half an ounce per hour, which is a very short half-life (length of effect) compared to other drugs—this is why one drink often leads to another.

How It Works: Alcohol is a *central nervous system depressant* that is rapidly absorbed from the stomach and small intestine into the bloodstream. From there it affects the brain and other cognitive and physical abilities (i.e. coordination and judgment). Alcohol affects every organ in the drinker's body and can damage a developing fetus. Continued drinking can increase risk of certain cancers, stroke, and liver disease. This brain damage or other effects can persist even if drinking ceases.

Usual Dose: A standard drink equals 0.6 ounces of pure ethanol, or 12 ounces of beer; 8 ounces of malt liquor, 5 ounces of wine or 1.5 ounces (a shot) of 80 proof distilled spirits of liquor (e.g. gin, rum, vodka or whisky).

Binge Drinking: One of the worst trends in alcohol use and abuse is binge drinking (also see **Section I**).

According to the National Institute of Alcohol Abuse and Alcoholism "binge drinking is pattern of drinking that is usually defined as a male consuming five or more drinks, and a woman consuming four or more drinks, in about 2 hours."

According to national surveys and the CDC, most binge drinkers are not actually alcohol-addicted and don't drink continually. Instead, the CDC reports these patterns as attributed to binge drinking.

- Approximately 92% of U.S. adults who drink excessively report binge drinking in the past 30 days.

- Although college students commonly binge drink, 70% of binge drinking episodes involve adults age 26 years and older.
- The prevalence of binge drinking among men is higher than the prevalence among women.
- Binge drinkers are 14 times more likely to admit to alcohol-impaired driving than non-binge drinkers.

- Binge drinking can be associated with cognitive deficits even among young drinkers.

- About 90% of the alcohol consumed by youth under the age of 21 in the United States is in the form of binge drinks.

- About 75% of the alcohol consumed by adults in the United States is in the form of binge drinks.

- The proportion of current drinkers who binge is highest in the 18- to 20-year-old group (51%).

- Alcohol dependence is highly inheritable and parents with family history need to pay special attention at all times.

Exactly What is Alcoholism? According to the National Institute on Alcohol Abuse and Alcoholism (NIAAA) "Alcoholism or alcohol dependence is a diagnosable disease characterized by a strong craving for alcohol, and/or continued use despite harm or personal injury. Alcohol abuse, which can lead to alcoholism, is a pattern of drinking resulting in harm to one's health, interpersonal relationships, or ability to work."

One final note on alcohol and alcohol addiction: Alcoholism is a chronic disease and it is important to understand that different people will experience different (any of a wide range) complications. An example of a chronic disease is diabetes, where one person experiences a complication such as vision loss, while another develops vascular disease leading to amputation. As you will see in the section on prescription drugs that follows, there are many other medications—especially over the counter drugs that contain alcohol and are easily abused without intending to do so.

One surprising and unintended roadblock for alcoholics is food cooked in alcohol. While it is widely thought that the alcohol in food cooks off, this is not true. There is actually enough to trigger the cravings that you may have experienced before rehab. There is an excellent, award winning book, *The Sober Kitchen* by Chef Liz Scott, published by Harvard Common Press and available in bookstores, amazon.com and on-line. This book explains this subject and also has hundreds of great recipes for a recovering alcoholic that focuses on "substitution" that provide just the same taste.

For more info visit The National Institute on Alcohol Abuse and Alcoholism (NIAAA) or the Centers For Disease Control (CDC).

Cocaine:

Today, it's often said, "there's nothing like coke". For thousands of years, indigenous populations in South America felt the same, but not over a soft drink. Then, chewing on the leaf of a small plant produced a source of energy and wellbeing. There wasn't a "drug scene" or rehab facilities but now all that has changed. Today the "scene" is about a drug called cocaine. No other illicit drug has ever burst so explosively onto the American scene. The carnage it has caused over the past 25 years has been responsible for an unprecedented increase in violent crime, injury, and economic impact. Among the worst effects of this disaster when it first occurred in the 1960's was the creation of an entire new middle class of addicted drug users aged 20-40.

Everyone knew their "office" dealers in the "cubby on the third floor", and thousands of people ended up in "high-end private rehabs" or those without resources often paid a worse price. At the root of the cocaine trade was an entire new group of "Drug Lords" who kept entire countries terrorized and at the same time made an unfathomable amount of money. Corruption was, and still is rampant in those countries.

Until cocaine resurfaced widely in the 1960's, very few people knew much about it. If they did it was in magazine articles like *National Geographic* and described as cultural phenomena, used in ceremonies and by the farmers to "clear their minds, elevate moods, help digestion, suppress appetite, increase longevity and fight altitude sickness." Drug abuse until then was largely driven by a generation of baby boomers looking to mellow out with marijuana at a rock concert or the musicians themselves. In fact, if you asked, most people would think coke was quasi-legal, even though it was classified illegal with major penalties and prison terms.

During the 60's and on into the 80's disco era, cocaine seemed to be everywhere, its effects perfect for the party-time lifestyle of most users. Relatively inexpensive, cocaine began to develop its own subculture that included rock stars, athletes, Wall Street executives, and the vast sums made were "washed" into real estate, condo projects and luxury living.

Like all good parties, it had to come to an end. It turned out that cocaine was not "safe" and like many stimulant drugs, led to addiction.

Cocaine, the powder, is neither a drug that appeared from thin air, nor has it been a significant part of ancient religious ceremonies. The plants that produce cocaine in their natural element, the eastern Andes mountains (Peru, Bolivia, Columbia), have always been a far more valuable cash crop than corn or wheat for the farmers. In fact, it is believed that cultivation may go back to 5000 BC or further.

Officially the plant is classified 'Erythroxylum Coca' and is grown between 500 to 1000 ft. above sea level. There are 250 plus species of coca plants but there are only two species with the active "coke" alkaloid.

COCAINE STREET NAMES Cocaine is also known as "blow, bump, C, candy, Charlies, crack, flake, rock, snow, toot".

Cocaine Through The Centuries: Archeologists also have found evidence going back to 1500 BC that the Incas used the coca plant then much as the native people do now, sucking on the leaves. It was not until the 14th and 15th centuries when the Spanish arrived in South America that the coca leaf was "discovered" and word trickled back to Europe and researchers there viewed it more with curiosity than a potential drug.

In 1855, a German scientist, Freidrich Gaedcke, isolated the chief alkaloid in the plant and named it cocaine. Quickly, word of its ability to numb the tongue spread and it was converted into a medicine and drug. However, cocaine swept the continent after a chemist, Angelo Marini, created an elixir that he called Vin Mariani and as an entrepreneur he literally went on the road to promote it, gathering endorsements from Thomas Edison, Pope Leo XIII and U.S. President William McKinley.

In another three decades, products containing cocaine were everywhere. An instant hit called Coca Cola appeared in 1886 and was one of the first products with cocaine to be sold in "drug" stores. The nickname Coke was a subtle suggestion of its active ingredient, but it worked and other odd products like the Coca Leaf Smoke Ball were "recommended by leading physicians."

By the turn of the 20th century, cocaine was being used more and more as a form of anesthesia and was a key aspect of the development of the neural blocking technique to enable surgery on specific parts of the body. About the same time, cocaine began to be used by small segments of the population many of whom were already into drug use, especially heroin, since it was thought to help quell withdrawal symptoms.

Like marijuana, when word of its danger began to surface, the American Pharmaceutical Association and other anti-drug crusaders included it in The Pure Food and Drug Act of 1906. By that time cocaine was no longer a part of many products like Coca Cola, but there have been controversies over the validity of this claim. As a result of the attention of law enforcement and more negative publicity (like Freud), cocaine slowly sank underground.

Many addiction specialists believe that the beginning of the end of the 1980's cocaine resurrection was smoking cocaine that gave you a greater and fast high. This was followed by crack, a crystallized form that changed the entire market perception of cocaine. Coke no longer "was it" but, instead turned deadly. Well-known athletes and multiple reports of death by crack OD's fueled the popular media outcries, along with TV and movies portraying coke dealers as corrupt Latin American dictators. Coke was no longer a party drug. The good news (see below) is that THE use of cocaine in any form has slowed considerably.

What Cocaine Does to You:

According to NIDA, cocaine is a powerfully addictive stimulant drug. It is a strong central nervous system stimulant that increases levels of dopamine, a brain chemical (or neurotransmitter) associated with pleasure, movement, motivation, euphoria, in the brain's reward circuit.

Certain brain cells, or neurons, use dopamine to communicate. Normally, dopamine is released by a neuron in response to a pleasurable signal (e.g., the smell of good food), and then recycled back into the cell that released it, thus shutting off the signal between neurons.

Cocaine acts by preventing the dopamine from being recycled, causing excessive amounts of the neurotransmitter to build up, amplifying the message to and response of the receiving neuron, and ultimately disrupting normal communication. It is this excess of dopamine that is responsible for cocaine's euphoric effects. With repeated use, cocaine can cause long-term changes in the brain's reward system and in other brain systems as well, which may eventually lead to addiction.

Tolerance to the cocaine high also often develops quickly. Many cocaine abusers report that they seek but fail to achieve as much pleasure as they did from their first exposure. Some users will increase their dose in an attempt to intensify and prolong the euphoria, but this can also increase the risk of adverse psychological or physiological effects.

Eventually a user may develop "cocaine sensitization" or "reverse tolerance". They may take less of the drug and have adverse undesirable affects such as paranoia and agitation. This phenomenon is a direct result of what could be called the drug memories and the result is often an agitated state.

Cocaine Is Abused In Many Ways:

Like most drugs of abuse, users seem to come up with more and more ways to use the drug to accommodate their preferences, hide the use and/or get the most for their money. Cocaine is a particular example of this:

Three routes of administration are commonly used for cocaine:

- Snorting is the process of inhaling cocaine powder through the nose, where it is absorbed into the bloodstream through the nasal tissues

- Injecting is the use of a needle to insert the drug directly into the bloodstream

- Smoking (either in powder as "freebase" or in "rock" form) called crack, involves inhaling cocaine vapor or smoke into the lungs, where absorption into the bloodstream is as rapid as it is by injection. (The powdered hydrochloride salt form of cocaine can be snorted or dissolved in water and then injected.)

(As discussed, cocaine leaves are often ingested but rarely out of its native environment in South America.)

Crack is the street name given to the form of cocaine that has been processed to make a rock crystal, which, when heated, produces vapors that are smoked. It appeared in urban areas in the mid-1980's when freebasing was popular. Unfortunately, freebase required use of ether and was unstable. Crack was created by using other ways to solidify the cocaine into a solid rock form. The term "crack" refers to the crackling sound produced by the rock as it is heated.

Crack is also seemingly less expensive than powder cocaine, but in reality is not, because its intense high sends the user back for more and more.

WARNING! All three methods of cocaine abuse can lead to addiction and other severe health problems, including increasing the risk of contracting HIV/AIDS and other infectious diseases.

What Is The Difference In Methods Of Use?

The intensity and duration of cocaine's effects—which include increased energy, reduced fatigue, and mental alertness—depend on the route of drug administration. The faster cocaine is absorbed into the bloodstream and delivered to the brain, the more intense the high. This is true of most drugs of abuse.

Injecting or smoking cocaine produces a quicker, stronger high than snorting. On the other hand, faster absorption usually means shorter duration of action: the high from snorting cocaine may last 15 to 30 minutes, but the high from smoking may last only 5 to 10 minutes. In order to sustain the high, a cocaine abuser has to administer the drug again. For this reason, cocaine is sometimes abused in binges—taken repeatedly within a relatively short period of time, at increasingly higher doses.

The difference between crack and powder cocaine is that crack creates a "high" in less than ten seconds instead of two minutes; it lasts less than 15 minutes. The effect is so quick because it goes directly from the lungs to the brain—creating a feeling of both a stimulant and anesthetic—the numb feeling in the throat is a hallmark of the effect.

Abusing cocaine has a variety of adverse effects on the body:

- Blood vessels constrict and can lead to coronary artery disease, heart attack, stroke and destruction of the smooth muscle.

- Pupils dilate

- Body temperature & heart rate rise

- Increased blood pressure

- Headaches

- Gastrointestinal complications (abdominal pain and nausea)

The Coke Diet? Famously, cocaine tends to decrease appetite and is sometimes used as a diet drug, however, chronic users can become malnourished as well.

Do different methods of use change side effects?

Yes. It's now very clear that different routes of use can change your risk:

- Continued snorting of cocaine leads to loss of the sense of smell, nosebleeds, problems with swallowing, hoarseness and a chronically runny nose.

- Ingesting cocaine can cause severe bowel gangrene as a result of reduced blood flow.

- Injecting cocaine can bring about severe allergic reactions and increased risk for contracting HIV/AIDS and other blood-borne diseases.

- Binge-patterned cocaine use may lead to irritability, restlessness, and anxiety.

- Cocaine abusers can also experience severe paranoia—a temporary state of full-blown paranoid psychosis—in which they lose touch with reality and experience auditory hallucinations.

- Functional brain imaging of cocaine addicts will show brain damage and can take 4-12 months of sustained abstinence for any recovery to show.

According to NIDA and multiple studies, no matter which method is used cocaine abusers are at higher risk for "acute cardiovascular or cerebrovascular emergencies, such as a heart attack or stroke, which may cause sudden death. Cocaine-related deaths are often a result of cardiac arrest or seizure, followed by respiratory arrest."

Use of multiple drugs is common among cocaine users, especially with another psychoactive drug. If coke and alcohol are combined, the body actually creates a new chemical within the body. With alcohol, the liver produces cocaethylene, and very intense euphoria.

Can You Get Off Coke?

Getting off cocaine or any addiction involves a variety of behavioral changes and these methods are described in the context of the person and abused drugs. All drug treatment has to be tailored to the person. However there are some methods that are common. These include an intense program of detoxification, medical treatment, social and family support, drug testing and also use of the 12-steps Alcoholics Anonymous approach.

While a priority, there are no medications, approved by the FDA for treatment; however there are multiple research studies underway. Most of these are aimed at relieving the cravings for cocaine and other esoteric drugs that can prevent cocaine from affecting the brain in the way it does now. In general, the behavioral programs with tough post-rehab drug testing seem to work best at this time.

Cocaine Data

Monitoring The Future Survey:

According to the 2009 Monitoring the Future survey—a national survey of eighth through twelfth-graders —there were continuing declines reported in the use of powder cocaine, with past-year usage levels reaching their lowest point since the early 1990s.

Significant declines in use were measured from 2008 to 2009 among 12th-graders across all three survey categories: lifetime use decreased from 7.2 percent to 6.0 percent; past-year use dropped from 4.4 percent to 3.4 percent; and past-month use dropped from 1.9 percent to 1.3 percent.

Survey measures showed other positive findings among

12th graders as well; their perceived risk of harm associated with powder cocaine use increased significantly during the same period. Additionally, survey participants in the 10th grade reported significant changes, with past-month use falling from 1.2 percent in 2008 to 0.9 percent in 2009.

National Survey on Drug Use and Health (NSDUH)

According to the 2008 National Survey on Drug Use and Health, the estimated percentage of persons aged 12 or older who used cocaine in the past month (0.7 percent) was similar to the percentage in 2007 and 2002. However, the percentage of past-month crack users in 2008 (0.1 percent of the population) was lower than in 2007 and all other years going back to 2002, with the exception of 2004.

From 2002 to 2008, rates of past-month cocaine use among youth aged 12 to 17 declined significantly, from 0.6 percent to 0.4 percent. Past-month cocaine use also dropped significantly among young adults aged 18 to 25 during this time period, from 2.0 percent to 1.5 percent.

Significant declines in the number or percentage of past-year cocaine initiates were also estimated among several age groups measured, including persons 12 or older and those aged 18 to 25. The percentage of past-year initiates also dropped significantly from 2007 to 2008 for crack use among the 12–17 age group.

Marijuana:

In **Section I**, marijuana, the most commonly abused illicit drug in the United States, is also discussed in some depth in the context of its thousands of years history as a controversial drug of choice for many. As socio-cultural phenomena, marijuana is significant to some and anathema to others. Critics characterize it as a dangerous substance that will drive users to crime, violence, wanton sexuality, and finally to madness. For generations others saw this plant as a valuable source of hemp fibers for clothing or other fabrics rather than a drug.

What are the facts? Is marijuana an "evil weed" that has strangled and corrupted countries or a potential useful substance for cancer pain and should IT be decriminalized? Is it as dangerous for adolescents as adults—or more?

MARIJUANA STREET NAMES:

Hashish: Boom, gangster, hash, hash oil

Marijuana: Blunt, dope, ganja, grass, herb, joint, bud, maryjane, pot, reefer, green, trees, smoke, sinsemilla, skunk, weed.

How Marijuana Is Used And Abused:

It is safe to say that marijuana is everywhere. According to the United Nations Office of Drugs and Crime, over 165 million people are regular users of marijuana or cannabis in another form such as hashish. It is certainly among the most widely used drugs in the world.

Marijuana is a dry, shredded green and brown mix of flowers, stems, seeds, and leaves derived from the hemp plant Cannabis sativa. The main active chemical in marijuana is delta-9-tetrahydrocannabinol, or THC for short. Marijuana is also used as the base of a more concentrated, resinous and powerful form of marijuana that is compressed into blocks called hashish.

Usually smoked as a hand rolled "cigarette" (known as a joint) or in a pipe, marijuana is also smoked in other forms to make it more powerful and there are many of these. One is called "blunts", which are cigars that have been emptied of tobacco and refilled with a mixture of marijuana and tobacco. This mode of delivery combines marijuana's active ingredients with nicotine and other harmful chemicals. Marijuana can also be mixed in food (ever hear about 'special' brownies?) or brewed as a tea.

"Marijuana smoke has a pungent and distinctive, usually sweet-and-sour odor. You only need to be exposed once to remember that smell".

How Does Marijuana Affect the Brain?

Scientists have learned a great deal about how THC acts in the brain to produce its many effects. When someone smokes marijuana, THC rapidly passes from the lungs into the bloodstream, which carries the chemical to the brain and other organs throughout the body.

THC acts upon specific sites in the brain, called cannabinoid receptors, kicking off a series of cellular reactions that ultimately lead to the "high" that users experience when they smoke marijuana. Some brain areas have many cannabinoid receptors; others have few or none. The highest density of cannabinoid receptors are found in parts of the brain that influence pleasure, memory, thinking, concentrating, sensory and time perception, and coordinated movement.

Not surprisingly, marijuana intoxication ("getting stoned" or "high") can cause:

- Perceptual distortion, causing accidents and injury

- Impaired coordination

- Difficulty thinking and problem solving

- Problems with learning and memory.

- Decreased reaction time

- Thwarted emotional development

- Social disruption

- Disorganization

- Psychosis (Schizophrenia and possible links)

Not surprisingly, several studies have found that drivers who were smoking marijuana were significantly impaired. These studies measured the amount of THC in drivers who caused accidents and they were found to be three to seven times more likely to be responsible for the accidents. There is no direct evidence that having previously smoked marijuana increases risk unless the driver is currently 'stoned' or 'high'.

Research has shown that, in chronic users, marijuana's adverse impact on learning and memory can last for days or weeks after the acute effects of the drug wears off. As a result, someone who smokes marijuana every day may be functioning at a suboptimal intellectual level all of the time.

Other studies into the effects of long-term cannabis use on the structure of the brain have yielded inconsistent results. It may be that the effects are too subtle for reliable detection by current techniques. A similar challenge arises in studies of the effects of chronic marijuana use on brain function. Brain imaging studies in chronic users tend to show some consistent alterations, but their connection to impaired cognitive functioning is far from clear. This uncertainty may stem from confounding factors such as other drug use, residual drug effects, or withdrawal symptoms in long-term chronic users.

The Marjuana Diet?

Unlike cocaine, marijuana users report that smoking pot increases all sensation, especially hunger which is usually called "the munchies". It is not uncommon to find marijuana users stretched out in front of the TV with buckets of popcorn and especially chocolate. It is not known to cause weight loss.

Can You Get Addicted To Pot?

Over time, marijuana abuse can lead to addiction; when defined as *compulsive drug seeking and abuse despite the known harmful effects upon functioning in the context of family, school, work, and recreational activities.*

Estimates suggest that about 9 percent of users become addicted to marijuana; this number increases among those who start young (to about 17 percent) and among daily users (25-50 percent).

Long-term marijuana abusers trying to quit report withdrawal symptoms including: irritability, sleeplessness, decreased appetite, anxiety, and drug craving, all of which can make it difficult to stop cravings. These symptoms begin within 1 day following abstinence, peak at 2-3 days, and subside within 1 or 2 weeks following drug cessation.

Can Marijuana Make You Crazy?

Unless you are genetically predisposed, it is not likely that marijuana will "make you crazy". A number of studies have shown an association between chronic marijuana use and increased rates of anxiety, depression, and schizophrenia. Some of these studies have shown age at first use to be an important risk factor, where early use is a marker of increased vulnerability to later problems. However, at this time, it is not clear whether marijuana use causes mental problems, exacerbates them, or reflects an attempt to self-medicate symptoms already in existence.

Chronic marijuana use, especially in a very young person, may also be a marker of risk for mental illnesses - including addiction - stemming from genetic or environmental vulnerabilities, such as early exposure to stress or violence. Currently, the strongest evidence links marijuana use and schizophrenia and/or related disorders. High doses of marijuana can produce an acute psychotic reaction; in addition, use of the drug may trigger the onset or relapse of schizophrenia in vulnerable individuals.

What Other Adverse Effects Does Marijuana Have on Health?

Heart: Marijuana increases heart rate by 20-100 percent shortly after smoking; this effect can last up to 3 hours. In one study, it was estimated that marijuana users have a 4.8-fold increase in the risk of heart attack in the first hour after smoking the drug.

Lungs: Numerous studies have shown marijuana smoke to contain carcinogens and to be an irritant to the lungs. In fact, marijuana smoke contains 50-70 percent more carcinogenic hydrocarbons than tobacco smoke. Marijuana users usually inhale more deeply and hold their breath longer than tobacco smokers do, which further increase the lungs' exposure to carcinogenic smoke. The link between marijuana smoking and cancers does remain unsubstantiated at this time. Nonetheless, marijuana smokers can have many of the same respiratory problems as tobacco smokers, such as daily cough and phlegm production, more frequent acute chest illness, and a heightened risk of lung infections.

What Treatment Options Exist?

Treatment options of marijuana use are similar to those described in the cocaine chapter although an individually tailored program is the most successful. The latest treatment data indicate that in 2008 marijuana accounted for 17 percent of admissions (322,000) to treatment facilities in the United States, second only to opiates among illicit substances. Marijuana admissions were primarily male (74 percent), Caucasian (49 percent), and young (30 percent were in the 12-17 age range). Those in treatment for primary marijuana abuse began use at an early age: 56 percent by age 14.

Is Marijuana Medicine?

This is a tricky question, especially in the context of thousands of years of use and also the fact that this has become as big a political issue as a medical question. As mentioned earlier in this book a number of states have passed their own laws like California where marijuana is the leading cash crop and sold openly.

Marijuana is not medicine and should not be used as such unless it meets the same standards that any other medication would before being approved by the FDA. It must establish efficacy in controlled studies.

Recommendations: The American Society of Addiction Medicine (ASAM), in a new "White Paper" lays out questions to be fully considered before medical marijuana would be approved. They say:

> *In order to think clearly about "medical marijuana," one must distinguish first between the therapeutic potentials of specific chemicals found in marijuana that are delivered in controlled doses by nontoxic delivery systems, and smoked marijuana.*

Second, one must consider the drug approval process in the context of public health, not just for medical marijuana but also for all medicines and especially for controlled substances. Controlled substances are drugs that have recognized abuse potential. Marijuana is high on that list because it is widely abused and a major cause of drug dependence in the United States and around the world. When physicians recommend use of scheduled substances, they must exercise great care. The current pattern of "medical marijuana" use in the United States is far from that standard.

If any components of marijuana are ever shown to be beneficial to treat any illness then those components can and should be delivered by nontoxic routes of administration in controlled doses just all other medicines are in the U.S.

ASAM asserts that cannabis, cannabis-based products, and cannabis delivery devices should be subject to the same standards that are applicable to other prescription medications and medical devices and that these products should not be distributed or otherwise provided to patients unless and until such products or devices have received marketing approval from the Food and Drug Administration.

ASAM rejects smoking as a means of drug delivery since it is not safe.

ASAM recognizes the supremacy of federal regulatory standards for drug approval and distribution. ASAM recognizes that states can enact limitations that are more restrictive but rejects the concept that states could enact more permissive regulatory standards. ASAM discourages state interference in the federal medication approval process.

ASAM rejects a process whereby State and local ballot initiatives approve medicines because these initiatives are being decided by individuals not qualified to make such decisions (based upon a careful science-based review of safety and efficacy, standardization and formulation for dosing, or provide a means for a regulated, closed system of distribution for marijuana which is a CNS drug with abuse potential).

ASAM recommends its members and other physician organizations and their members reject responsibility for providing access to cannabis and cannabis-based products until such time that these materials receive marketing approval from the Food and Drug Administration.

Scientists continue to investigate the medicinal properties of THC and other cannabinoids to better evaluate and harness their ability to help patients suffering from a broad range of conditions, while avoiding the adverse effects of smoked marijuana.

Marijuana Data:

National Survey on Drug Use and Health (NSDUH):

According to the National Survey on Drug Use and Health, in 2009, 16.7 million Americans aged 12 or older used marijuana at least once in the month prior to being surveyed, an increase over the rates reported in all years between 2002 and 2008. There was also a significant increase among youth aged 12-17, with current use up from 6.7 percent in 2008 to 7.3 percent in 2009, although this rate is lower than what was reported in 2002 (8.2 percent). Past-month use also increased among those 18-25, from 16.5 percent in 2008 to 18.1 percent in 2009.

Monitoring the Future Survey:

Results from the 2009 Monitoring the Future survey show, as in the past few years, a stall in the decline of marijuana use that began in the late 1990s among our nation's youth. As discussed above, one important and key aspect of prevention is perception of danger and also *availability.*

According to the 2010 Monitoring the Future survey "*perceived availability*" is measured by the question "How difficult do you think it would be for you to get each of the following types of drugs, if you wanted some?" Answer categories are "probably impossible," "very difficult," "fairly difficult," "fairly easy," and "very easy." For 8th and 10th graders, an additional answer category—"can't say, drug unfamiliar"—is offered and included in the calculations

In 2009, 11.8 percent of 8th-graders, 26.7 percent of 10th-graders, and 32.8 percent of 12th-graders reported past-year use. In addition, perceived risk of marijuana use declined among 8th- and 10th-graders, and disapproval of marijuana use declined among 10th-graders. This is a concern because changes in attitudes and beliefs often drive changes in drug use.

The most important specific use findings to emerge from the Monitoring The Future 2010 survey reflect the falling "perception of marijuana risk" is tied to an escalation of "initiating drug use" among adolescents.

Marijuana use, which had been rising among teens for the past two years, continued to rise in 2010 in all prevalence periods for all three grades. This stands in stark contrast to the long, gradual decline that had been occurring over the preceding decade.

Of relevance, perceived risk for marijuana has been falling in recent years. Of particular relevance, daily marijuana use increased significantly in all three grades in 2010; and stands at 1.2%, 3.3%, and 6.1% in grades 8, 10, and 12.

In other words, nearly one in sixteen high school seniors today is a current daily, or near-daily, marijuana user.

Marijuana is by far the most prevalent drug included in the any illicit drug use index, an increase in prevalence occurred for that index as well as for marijuana. The proportions using any illicit drug other than marijuana had been declining gradually since about 2001, but no further decline occurred in 2010.

Other Information Sources

For additional information on marijuana, please visit www. marijuana-info.org. and the National Institutes for Drug Abuse (www.nida.gov.)

Prescription Medications

It would not be an exaggeration to say that "Prescription Drugs" have been around forever—depending on your definition of a prescription drug. Going back, perhaps as far as civilization exists, someone in some tribe was designated as the person to go see when you were sick. This could mean a "holy man" who had discovered a potion with herbs or leaves or someone a few centuries later who could read and write and follow medical texts left by civilizations going back to 5000 B.C.

These ancient people were right about the best source of what we have come to call a prescription drug. What is the most fascinating aspect of the evolution of prescription drugs (and others) is that many actually do come from trees, plants and other vegetation. Today, about 120 different "distinct chemical substances" from plants now account for about 25 % of all drugs. Of those that are natural, many have synthetic versions spun off to manufacture in large quantities.

This evolution has led to standardization of the production process. Each country today is supposed to carefully oversee the testing and use of prescription drugs, but often the nature of the active substance in the drug determines this. For example, Germany monitors an herbal-based product as a prescription drug, while in the US we sell the same medicine, but it has a certain amount of the active substance taken out and we call it an "extract" and it's sold openly without prescriptions in stores everywhere.

A classic example of this natural discovery is *quinine* that was already saving thousands, but after being created artificially, it now saves millions. More than a century ago, a chemical was discovered in the rain forest in the bark of a tree called *Chinchona ledgeriana* and the chemical that resulted in quinine was extracted. When processed it was discovered that quinine could treat malaria. Malaria had been known for over 50,000 years. Unfortunately, it took decades for anyone to even understand that the source of this disease was a mosquito that liked human flesh, but was infested by a deadly parasite that liked the bug just as much.

The breakthrough with quinine came when scientists were able to "copy" or synthesize the chemical from the bark, reducing the need for overuse of the tree. This may seem relatively unimportant in an age where vaccines protect us from many diseases that have swept across continents leaving millions dead. In fact, there were only 1500 cases of malaria in the US in 2008. However, in 2008 there were between 190,000,000—311,000,000 cases reported and 1,100,000 fatalities in countries with poor health and hygiene or no medical care and/or in geographic areas where the insects live.

Over time the chinchona tree also provided more than a cure for malaria, when it was discovered that the bark also produced *quinidine* and could be used in the treatment of heart conditions. It has not been synthesized yet, but is sold under a number of brands. Some of the more familiar drug names with plant sources are:

- Digoxin (Digitalis plant)

- Codeine & Morphine (Papaver sonniferin)

- L-Dopa (Mucuna sp)

- Ephederine (Ephdra sinica)

- Nicotine-used as insectiside (Nicotiana tabacum)

- Theophylline (Theobroma cacao)

The National Cancer Institute (NCI), searching among the more than 250,000 plant species on the planet, is finding one of the most important uses of plants is as sources of medication. According to NCI more than 50% of these plants are hidden in the rain forests and spread around the world. Several new medications derived from plants have FDA approval and have shown high levels of effectiveness fighting leukemia and various tumors.

What Is A Prescription Drug Today?

Today's prescription drugs are technically referred to as extemporaneous prescriptions which means that it's written for you, for a specific acute need and given to you for immediate use. Other prescription drugs are those prescribed for a chronic illness. There are also "compound" drugs that are actually "mixed" in the pharmacy by the pharmacist.

The concept of a prescription has changed completely over the past century and is continuing to evolve. Initially, medications were created by hucksters selling patent medicine, awarding the "honorary

MD's" to themselves. Fortunately this changed in the 20th century when physicians and legitimate pharmaceutical companies were licensed and regulated.

Standardizing the medications we take has also made more and more medications available and according to the Department of Health and Human Service we each take at least one prescription a year and one in six take three. Life expectancy is up and chronic diseases like cardiovascular problems, cancer, and stroke have slowed. There is no question that our overall health and longevity has increased, but the expense for both patients and the government programs has also skyrocketed.

Prescription Drug Dangers: The Bad News

Despite all the benefits we derive from medications, especially for chronic conditions and related problems such as pain relief, certain prescription medications have become a danger and now occupy their own category as a potentially addictive substance. The risk to adolescents with developing brains is particularly critical and growing numbers of junior high and high school students are abusing medications from virtually every category.

NIDA reported that in 2009, 16 million people over age 12 have used a tranquilizer, stimulant, or sedative for nonmedical purposes.

Prescription drug abuse has increased in virtually every category and it is now an epidemic that has gained the attention of the Federal Government that has launched plans to significantly increase education and law enforcement efforts. According to statistics released by a joint U.S. Government task force in April 2011 "prescription drug abuse is our Nation's fastest-growing drug problem."

The number of people who have unintentionally overdosed on prescription drugs now exceeds the number who overdosed during the crack cocaine epidemic of the 1980's and the black tar heroin epidemic of the 1970's combined. In 2007, approximately 27,000 people died from unintentional drug overdoses, driven mostly by prescription drugs.

Additionally, according to the Substance Abuse and Mental Health Services Administration, the number of Americans in 2009 aged 12 and older currently abusing pain relievers has increased by 20% since 2002. Further, visits by individuals to hospital emergency rooms involving the misuse or abuse of pharmaceutical drugs have doubled over the past five years.

"Unintentional drug overdose is a growing epidemic in the US and is now the leading cause of injury death in 17 states," CDC Director Dr. Thomas Frieden says."

The Most Abused Prescription Drugs:

There are three basic categories of prescription medication:

1 **Opioids**—strong painkillers

2 **CNS—Depressants (anxiolytics and sedatives)**—To treat and prevent anxiety and sleep disorders/aids through the central nervous system.

3 **Stimulants (psychostimulants)**—treats sleep disorders, increased alertness, attention deficit disorders and a number of other conditions based on the patient's age and health or psychological disorders.

Opioids: This group of prescription drugs can either be of great benefit or create a never ending loop becoming addictive in the traditional sense or seeking to repeat use without regard for the consequences. The main reason a doctor will prescribe an opioid is a need to relieve serious chronic or acute pain. The use maybe legitimate in the beginning and for real pain, but if the brain responds and "likes opiates" it goes beyond pain relief. The person and the brain like it and that creates a reinforcing relief of psychic pain providing a sense of well being.

Patients describe this as more than a euphoric or a warm and fuzzy feeling. Other things in their life "are better" and they feel a sort of numbing—not only a high. Some people are sedated and others get energized with high levels of energy. For example, opioids are used for patients after operations, for chronic pain like rheumatoid arthritis, dental surgery and while recovering from an accident. They are highly effective as a painkiller, but also dangerous if proper dosage is not followed.

Opioids, because they are so powerful are regarded as narcotics. (Other opioids include heroin, and opium, but are not prescription drugs and are described on. Only recently has use of both Vicodin and OxyContin increased among adolescents, but now perceived availability has gone up without a clear perception of risk to temper abuse among teenagers.

Medications in this class:

- Vicodin (hydrocodone)

- OxyContin (oxycodone an oral, controlled-release dose)

- Morphine and Fentanyl (for severe pain i.e. cancer)

- Fentanyl, codeine, Darvon (propoxyphene), Dilaudid (hydromorphone), Demerol (meperidine), Lomotil (diphenoxylate) for milder pain, coughs, and diarrhea.

How Opioids Work & Are Used:

In each of our brains, spinal cords and GI tracts there are proteins called "opioid receptors." When you take an opioid it attaches to these proteins and changes the way they have been affecting us— for example shutting down our perception of the pain, effectively blocking it. Opioids can also affect the pleasure centers in our brain with a boost of euphoria but it is short lasting. Repeated abuse of opioids can lead to addiction quite easily.

Since most opioids can be taken orally as a pill or tablet they are also frequently crushed and snorted—or possibly "cooked down" to a liquid base and snorted or injected. This method also leads to many deaths by overdose since drugs like OxyContin are supposed to be long acting. If snorted or injected the release into the bloodstream is quick and intense, causing overdose and heart failure from respiratory arrest.

Opioids cause several other reactions or adverse effects even when used properly. Like many other drugs they create drowsiness, gastrointestinal problems and even breathing problems, which is why you must follow the prescribed dosages exactly. Additionally, these drugs are very dangerous when combined with alcohol, antihistamines, barbiturates, or tranquilizers known as benzodiazepines.

Always follow your doctor's orders when taking opioids and make sure you let your physician know that you are on one of these medications.

What You Can Do To Stop Opioid Abuse:

You may not be addicted to opioids, but if you are using opioids beyond what your physician prescribes, you are likely *dependent*. In fact, this is an actual physical dependence. What has happened is that your body has adapted to the pain killing benefits of the drug that has led to *tolerance* which basically means you need more and more to feel the same relief.

If you are taking an opioid, just as you should not use them without supervision of a doctor, do not stop abruptly without medical supervision. You may experience muscle and bone pain, insomnia, GI upset, cold flashes and restless leg movement among other symptoms as you discontinue the drug.

Treating opioid addiction (including heroin use) will always be part of a good comprehensive program including detoxification, therapy, behavioral modification, attending twelve step meetings, and one of several medications that have been effective in reducing the desire for more of these drugs. The effectiveness of these drugs is directly related to compliance by the patient and matching the correct medication to the patient's circumstances. The goal is to put in place a program based on the "harm reduction" goal.

There are three major medications used in opioid treatment as part of the treatment plan described above:

- **Methadone,** the best known to most, is a synthetic opioid that eliminates withdrawal symptoms and relieves craving. It has been commonly used for more than 30 years to treat people addicted to heroin as well as opiates. Methadone is dispensed on a daily basis at a specially licensed clinic directly to the patient. This can cause problems for patients who are not located near a methadone center. There can be unintended side effects including respiratory effects.

- The three drugs that follow are easier to administer and to create compliance because they are administered in a physician's office and the doctor can monitor the patient closely.

- **Buprenorphine** is also a synthetic opioid that is being used for heroin and opioid addiction. It is also used in treatment of withdrawal. Known as a partial agonist, it does not have the full blocking effect on opiate receptors thus Buprenorphine is less reinforcing and unlikely to cause addiction. Rarely does it cause respiratory compromise unless combined with another CNS depressant drug like a benzodiazepine. It can be prescribed in a physician's office as an injection, wearable patch, pills or a sublingual patch. It is considered safer than methadone causing less respiratory compromise.

- **Naltrexone** is a long-acting opioid blocker that can be part of a relapse prevention program and approved in use of an alcohol relapse program although it has not been as successful as other agonist blockers. It also is a deterrent for opiate abuse. This medication cannot be used until detoxification is complete to avoid strong withdrawal symptoms. It is administered orally or injected.

- **Naloxone** is a short acting opioid receptor blocker that works by binding to the opiate receptors and blocking opiates from binding to receptors.

- **Suboxone** is a sublingual narcotic medication also used for the treatment of opioid dependence but must be carefully supervised by a physician. It is, like the other drugs, available only by prescription, and must be taken under a doctor's care as prescribed. It is a combination of buprenorphine and naloxone. It prevents the effects of bupenorphine if injected. It is available as a patch or film.

- **Naloxone** is a short-acting opioid receptor blocker that works similarly as the others above and is effective treating overdoses. It is only used through injection.

CNS—Depressants:

Central Nervous System Depressants (CNS) are targeted at multiple mood disorders in various strengths and brands. Called psychotherapeutic drugs, they create a serious risk for dependence and addiction when abused.

Most people today are commonly prescribed these drugs when they are having mild to severe psychological problems such as anxiety, problems sleeping, sadness and simply feeling that day-to-day coping at work or home is too difficult. In general they are combined with some sort of psychological therapy and intended for short time use. CNS depressants most often prescribed are *sedatives* and *tranquilizers* from the group known as *benzodiazepines*—the best known are Valium and Xanax. These are also among the most abused and recognized by adolescents.

How Do CNS Drugs Affect Your Brain?

CNS medication actually slows your brain function (and some are used as an anesthetic). They are classified as three different groups even though they work similarly. They are designed to increase the action of a specific neurotransmitter known as gamma-aminobutyric acid (GABA). The neurotransmitter is a key chemical in the brain that enables our cells to communicate, sending messages, in this case to slow or decrease brain activity. This is the common thread to increase GABA activity and delivers a calmness or even sleep.

These drugs are divided into three groups, based on their chemistry and pharmacology:

- *Barbiturates*, such as mephobarbital (Mebaral) and sodium pentobarbital (Nembutal), are used as preanesthetics, promoting sleep.

- *Benzodiazepines*, such as diazepam (Valium), alprazolam (Xanax), Klonopin (clonazepam) can be prescribed to treat anxiety spectrum disorders-including general anxiety, panic and phobias, event-specific anxiety, acute stress reactions, panic attacks, acute convulsions, and sleep disorders. For the latter, benzodiazepines are usually prescribed only for short-term relief of sleep problems because of the development of tolerance and risk of addiction. When used for anxiety is it combined with a benzodiazepine and an SSRI like Prozac or Zoloft. The benzodiazepine is tapered off when the SSRI's go into full effect.

Benzodiazapines are often used with by a person who combines another drug or alcohol. Any indication of this in a family history is a sure sign that there is the presence of history risk factor.

Benzodiazapines can cause falls, memory problems, car accidents, intoxications, and worsening depression. Do not stop taking these medications abruptly or without supervisor of a physician.

According to Robert L. DuPont, M.D., former Director of The National Institute of Drug Abuse, rarely do you create an escalating need for benzodiazapines. The dose that works will also relieve anxiety—if you need more you're in trouble and are developing addictive symptoms.

- Newer sleep medications, such as zolpidem (Ambien), zaleplon (Sonata), and eszopiclone (Lunesta), are now more commonly prescribed to treat sleep disorders. These medications are non-benzodiazepines that act at a subset of the benzodiazepine receptors and appear to have a lower risk for abuse and addiction. Although they have a lower risk for abuse and addiction they still have some potential liability.

Warning

CNS depressants are usually taken orally, sometimes in combination with other drugs or to counteract the effects of other legal or illicit drugs (e.g., stimulants).

CNS depressants should not be combined with any medication or substance that causes drowsiness, including prescription pain medicines, certain OTC cold and allergy medications, and alcohol. If combined, they can slow both heart rate and respiration, which can be fatal.

CNS Addiction and Abuse:

Any medications that affect the brain and change behavior like anxiety and stress or vital functions like sleep can create tolerance and dependence over time. Some will create an addictive pattern more rapidly depending on dose and sensitivity of the receptor sites. Despite their benefits, they can be dangerous if not taken exactly as prescribed. **In addition, it's very important to report any side effects or problems to your physician as soon as they appear.**

Abruptly stopping use of CNS medication can be very dangerous. The brain's activity has been slowed by the CNS and when it stops, it can "rebound" and cause seizures as the brain "reboots". **Do not discontinue any CNS medication without the supervision of your physician.**

Treating CNS Addiction: In addition to medical supervision during withdrawal, counseling in an inpatient or outpatient setting can help people who are overcoming addiction to CNS depressants. It's critical that the patient is tapered off the medication and transferred slowly to another appropriate, non-addictive drug. This is followed by cognitive-behavioral therapy that has been used successfully to help individuals in treatment for abuse of benzodiazepines.

This type of therapy focuses on modifying a patient's thinking, expectations, and behaviors while simultaneously increasing his or her skills for coping with various life issues and most importantly help develop non-pharmaceutical solutions to avoid past behavior. This is the best way to use "talk therapy" to develop coping strategies. It's often very helpful to have a spiritual component like a 12-step program.

Stimulants:

Each drug in this class is distinct, but in general they elevate mood, temporarily increase feelings of well-being, energy, awareness, and improve concentration. As stimulant "drugs" they all have similar neurologic properties and effects in the brain: **Psychostimulants**

- Caffeine

- Nicotine

- Cocaine

- Methyphenadate: (Ritalin, Concerta)

- Amphetamines: (Dexedrine) (Atterral)

- Others psychostimulant: (Provigial, Phentremine, Vivands)

How Do Prescription Stimulants Affect the Brain?

All stimulants work by primarily increasing dopamine norepinephrine levels in the brain. Dopamine is a brain chemical (or neurotransmitter) associated with pleasure, movement, and attention. The therapeutic effect of stimulants is achieved by slow and steady increases of dopamine, which are similar to the natural production of the chemical by the brain. The doses prescribed by physicians start low and increase gradually until a therapeutic effect is reached. However, when taken in doses and routes other than those prescribed, stimulants can increase brain dopamine in a rapid and highly amplified manner—as do most other drugs of abuse— disrupting normal communication between brain cells, producing euphoria, and increasing the risk of addiction.

Stimulants And Your Brain:

Everyone has many common chemical structures in the brain called neurotransmitters. Two are dopamine and norepinephrine. All stimulants work by increasing dopamine levels in the brain— dopamine is a brain chemical (or neurotransmitter) associated with pleasure, movement, and attention

Dopamine is important in brain reward, motivation and movement and to some degree attention. The stimulant drug's job is to slowly increase—called the therapeutic dose—to the proper effect. This is how they are normally released without a drug. If too little is sensed by the brain, it fails to get its "reward." However, if too much is taken or the drug uses an "alternate" route to the brain the body will respond to the effect with the surge associated with addiction.

If you take any stimulant in any manner other than the gradual approach your physician has prescribed, you'll find yourself in danger. Your body can't stay that way disrupting normal communication between brain cells, producing euphoria, agitation, paranoia, overstimulation, psychosis and increased the risk of addiction.

Stimulants and ADHD

ADHD or attention-deficit hyperactivity disorder is a legitimate disorder, usually appearing in children who are about 6-7, just entering school. It's estimated that 8 percent of children ages 4–17 and 2.9–4.4 percent of adults have ADHD. There is a 2:1 male to female ratio in this disorder, meaning that twice as many males are found to have ADHD.

It's likely that a child may exhibit the classic symptoms; lack of attention or inability to keep focused (needs constant redirection to task), hyperactive (can't sit still), impulsive (acts before thinking) and very distractible. Often this behavior creates chaos in the school environment, but if it goes undiagnosed, then the child falls behind in school. The child may be mislabeled as a goof-off, slacker (lazy), or a troublemaker. In adolescence the problem may appear to slowly disappear; however, the experts now believe that an ADHD child becomes an ADHD adult – the difference being that the symptoms change (hyperactivity morphs into fidgeting, finger-tapping, etc.) as the adult learns coping strategies. An ADHD adult may be constantly late, disorganized (messy), tends to procrastinate, forgets appointments, commitments, deadlines, is constantly losing or misplacing things (like keys, wallet, bills, etc.) and is easily overwhelmed by responsibilities. Many adults with ADHD learn to live with the condition or channel it into energy for school or work.

Attention Deficit Disorder (ADD) is a subset of ADHD. The difference is that the symptoms are not exactly the same. Those with ADD do not manifest hyperactivity, but instead are generally inattentive and demonstrate an inability to focus or concentrate. These children are often labeled "day-dreamers" by teachers.

What Is the Role of Stimulants in the Treatment of ADHD?

It is very, very important to ensure that the diagnosis of ADHD or ADD is correct and not an alternative problem like depression, anxiety, something physiological or even drug use. It has been shown that a complete work-up and evaluation should be performed before any medication is considered. There is evidence also, that people who use psychostimulant drugs have higher rates of drug abuse and addiction, so drug testing should also be part of the evaluation.

The use of stimulants as part of therapy for ADHD is controversial for several reasons. One, of course, is that care should always be taken when a medication is prescribed for any child and everyone agrees on that. The second is that there are people who believe that giving stimulants to a child or adolescent may lead to a later risk of substance abuse. There is no evidence that this is true and multiple studies show that if the medication is taken as prescribed and when, there is little risk—but we do believe that research should be continuing.

One thing to keep in mind is that a child or adolescent with ADHD may not receive the full benefits of their education, may develop social problems since they have trouble with group activities, and may develop low self esteem and other mental health issues. Any child with suspected ADHD at any age should be evaluated thoroughly, especially if cognitive and family problems are growing visible. Use of stimulants and a program of therapy can alleviate many of the problems described above.

Most Frequently Prescribed Stimulants For ADHD:

- Amphetamines (e.g., Adderall, a mix of amphetamine salts) are the most popular drugs for ADHD but they also have a high street value and are sold

- Vivance is called a pro-drug meaning by itself it metabolizes, so more and more of it used and it quickly converts to dexedrine

- Methylphenidate (e.g., Ritalin and Concerta, a formulation that releases medication in the body over a period of time. Concerta has less of a street value.)

- These medications have what is called a "paradoxically calming" or "assist in focusing" effect on individuals with ADHD. Studies show that because methylphenidate increases the release of dopamine, it can improve attention and focus in individuals who have dopamine "signals" that are not providing enough feedback. If an ADHD/ADD child is put on a proper course of medication, it can turn their lives around.

Why Stimulants Are Abused:

It's critical to remember that for stimulants to be both effective and safe, they have to be taken as prescribed. Sometimes called the "steroids of studying" by medical and law students because they help withstand long hours, often they are abused because people believe they can increase both their physical and mental performances.

This is not true, because eventually they cause adverse effects like increased blood pressure, heart rate, body temperature, and decrease sleep and appetite. When used as an appetite suppressant it can lead to malnutrition and its consequences. Repeated use of stimulants can lead to feelings of hostility and paranoia. At high doses, they can lead to serious cardiovascular complications, including stroke.

One drug called Provigil is used to enhance wakefulness-counteracting the effect of benzodiazapines used at night by those who also have to be awake during the day.

Stimulants can also, when used improperly, become a true risk especially when broken down to powders or injected, leading to an uncontrolled rise in dopamine and possible overdose. If continual use at high doses are abruptly stopped, withdrawal including fatigue, depression, and disturbed sleep patterns are possible.

Prescription Stimulant Drug Data:

Monitoring the Future Survey:

Each year, the Monitoring the Future (MTF) survey assesses the extent of drug use among 8th-, 10th-, and 12th-graders nationwide. For amphetamines and methylphenidate, the survey measures only past-year use, which refers to use at least once during the year preceding an individual's response to the survey. Use outside of medical supervision was first measured in the study in 2001; nonmedical use of stimulants has been falling since then, with total declines between 25 percent and 42 percent at each grade level surveyed. MTF data for 2008 indicate past-year nonmedical use of Ritalin by 1.6 percent of 8th-graders, 2.9 percent of 10th-graders, and 3.4 percent of 12th-graders.

Since its peak in the mid-1990s, annual prevalence of amphetamine use fell by one-half among 8th-graders to 4.5 percent and by nearly one-half among 10th-graders to 6.4 percent in 2008. Amphetamine use peaked somewhat later among 12th-graders and has fallen by more than one-third to 6.8 percent by 2008. Although general nonmedical use of prescription stimulants is declining in this group, when asked, "What amphetamines have you taken during the last year without a doctor's orders?" 2.8 percent of all 12th-graders surveyed in 2007 reported they had used Adderall. Amphetamines rank third among 12th-graders for past-year illicit drug use.

Other Information Sources

For more information on treating ADHD, visit the Web site for the National Institute of Mental Health, National Institutes of Health, at www.nimh.nih.gov.

For street terms searchable by drug name, street term, cost and quantities, drug trade, and drug use, visit www.whitehousedrugpolicy. gov/.

Methamphetamine:

Methamphetamine or **meth, is a CNS stimulant** that is similar chemically to amphetamines. It is so dangerous that is now classified as a Schedule II drug and is only available through a doctor.

- Meth's medical uses are limited, and only rarely used and in limited dosages

- In general, meth comes from labs hidden in basements or rural areas. The labs are volatile, often exploding and wiping away an entire block

- Meth is also smuggled into this Country by foreign drug rings

- A white crystal powder, meth is dissolved in water or alcohol, injected, snorted and smoked

Meth and Your Brain

Methamphetamine acts similarly to other CNS drugs by raising the levels of dopamine and blocking receptor sites. The critical difference is that the unregulated level can have a catastrophic effect. Its ability to release dopamine rapidly in reward regions of the brain produces the intense euphoria, or "rush," that many users feel after snorting, smoking, or injecting the drug. It's extremely dangerous because its effects can linger for a lengthy period.

Over time, continued use of meth actually affects the brain structure and functions such as motor skills and learning ability along with memory. Even without continually using meth, its effects can last for more than a year before the brain rebuilds.

The effect of meth is not only dose-related, but can be similar to other stimulants including inability to sleep, no appetite, rapid heartbeat, elevated pulse and sweating. Chronic use can create paranoid vision psychosis, violent behavior and delusions. The classic meth user is often portrayed as writhing on the floor swatting insects attacking—which may actually be what they are seeing. Malnutrition can set in with likely side effects such as dental problems sometimes called "meth mouth."

Meth and HIV

Meth users are known to have high rates of HIV/AIDS and Hepatitis B&C rates. The reason is simple, meth's pull is so strong that many abusers do not practice safe sex nor do they use clean or sterile needles if they are injecting. Brain damage among meth users can also increase the progression of HIV/AIDS

Can You Get Off Meth?

The typical treatment for meth addiction is similar to the other models used with other drugs in this section and combining cognitive behavior interventions and behavioral therapy; counseling for addicts and family, 12-step programs and drug testing. There are no medications at this time approved to treat methamphetamine addiction.

Meth Data

Monitoring the Future Survey

Methamphetamine use among teens appears to have dropped significantly in recent years, according to data revealed by the 2009 Monitoring the Future survey. The number of high-school seniors reporting past-year use is now only at 1.2 percent, which is the lowest since questions about methamphetamine were added to the survey in 1999; at that time, it was reported at 4.7 percent. Lifetime use among 8th-graders was reported at 1.6 percent in 2009, down significantly from 2.3 percent in 2008. In addition, the proportion of 10th-graders reporting that crystal methamphetamine was easy to obtain has dropped to 14 percent, down from 19.5 percent 5 years ago.

National Survey on Drug Use and Health

According to the 2008 National Survey on Drug Use and Health, the number of past-month methamphetamine users age 12 and older decreased by over half between 2006 and 2008. Current (past-month) users were numbered at 731,000 in 2006, 529,000 in 2007, and 314,000 in 2008. Significant declines from 2002 and 2008 also were noted for lifetime and past-year use in this age group.

From 2002 to 2008, past-month use of methamphetamine declined significantly among youths aged 12 to 17, from 0.3 percent to 0.1 percent, and young adults aged 18 to 25 also reported significant declines in past-month use, from 0.6 percent in 2002 to 0.2 percent in 2008.

Other Information Resources:

For more information on methamphetamine abuse and addiction, visit www.drugabuse.gov/drugpages/methamphetamine.html.

To find publicly funded treatment facilities by state, visit www.findtreatment.samhsa.gov.

For street terms searchable by drug name, street term, cost and quantities, drug trade, and drug use, visit www.whitehousedrugpolicy.gov/streetterms/default.asp.

Over-The-Counter Drugs:

Over-the-Counter drugs (OTC)—anything available without a prescription that you buy in a dedicated pharmacy or any other store that sells anything from analgesics to groceries have become a sort of corner drug dealer for the current adolescent and college generations. For these groups, traditional street drugs are old school and costly.

Unfortunately, many of these drugs and their effects can be as lethal as stimulants or binge drinking—but much easier to obtain and sometimes even "on sale" in a big box store. Over the past two to three decades the nature of OTCs has changed. Until then the use of OTC's was primarily a desperation drug for alcoholics. Most effective cough syrups were part alcohol and often produced a mild buzz.

Today, OTC's are now a recreational drug used primarily by teenagers, and as use has increased so have accidental deaths and dozens of overdoses. The worst aspect of teen OTC drug use is that unlike other drugs profiled above, they do not perceive the same level of danger that they see in other drugs. The reasons are obvious:

- Teens use these drugs to get a buzz or stay awake in school

- They can get them down the street in a store, on the internet or even in the family medicine cabinet. Teens (56%) think it is easy to get an OTC

- They are also conditioned to the safety of OTCs since they have been doled out at home since they were kids

- Safety is not a real perceived problem

- 40% feel OTCs are much safer than illegal drugs

- 31% are OK with occasional use of OTCs

- 55% do not feel that abusing cough medicine is dangerous and 10% do just that

There are several main OTC products that are abused:

- Cough and cold medicines

- Motion sickness drugs

- Inhalants

- Floor cleaners

- Diet Pills

- Analgesics

- Sleep Aids

DXM Drives The Trend:

Over 100 cough and cold medicines have a key chemical called **Dextromethorphan** or **DXM.** These include popular and highly promoted brands like Robitussin, NyQuil, Vicks Formula 44 and Coricidin HBP—all well known and most children and adults have used one or more and usually safely.

Drugs such as Robitussin, NyQuil, Vicks Formula 44, and Coricidin HBP Cough and Cold tablets contain a chemical called Dextromethorphan (DXM), which is found in more than 120 non-prescription cough and cold medications. DXM is the ingredient in these products that have been leading the OTC crisis. The teens call them by nicknames that you've probably never heard including *Robo, Skittles, Triple C's, Dex, Vitamin D, and Tussin.*

Some contain greater DXM (i.e. Coricidin HBP Cough and Cold tablets) and of course are stronger and pack a potent punch. Since Coricidin is a tablet (i.e. Skittles) it makes getting high easier than drinking cough syrup—which you can remember was not tasty when you were a kid.

DXM did not appear in our cough and cold products until the mid-1970's when it was thought that adding DXM (a synthetic similar to morphine) would make it more effective. The combination did strengthen the drug but also created a strong word of mouth about its abuse potential. When overdoses began to appear—often among groups in a single school, drug stores and other outlets controlled sales by putting it behind the counter, requiring some authority to permit sales and limiting how much can be sold.

The DXM Effect:

Dextromethorphan is *usually* a safe and effective cough suppressant, when taken as directed. Since DXM doses are rarely the same, and its effects change with each time it is used. Abusing DXM leads to depression and possible hallucinations. It can be mildly stimulating or distort vision ("stoned"). Too much DXM causes impaired judgment, lack of physical coordination, gastrointestinal upset and loss of balance. Driving, swimming and any activity that requires judgment will be compromised.

Shockingly, DXM can be purchased as bulk powder on the Internet and there are actually web sites that offer hints for "a better high."

Talking With Your Family:

OTC- proofing your home is a combination of both common sense and vigilance and, honestly, a small dose of worry utilized in a rational manner will also give your child an opportunity to have a two-way conversation. Still, most parents have a feeling of responsibility and headlines or talking with friends can raise red flags, even when not valid. Here are a few common questions and some suggestions from NIDA that have proven helpful:

Is My Child Abusing DXM?

If your child seems to like the taste of the cough product recommended too much or continues to take it when they are recovered—this is a signal.

If the medicine cabinet is empty—and cough syrup was a staple, you are justified in asking about it or even checking in his or her room or backpack.

Time For A Talk:

Even with a few signs of use, talking sooner rather than later is called for:

- Make sure you and your child are talking the same language—let them know you are informed on the dangers of the use of all OTCs and discuss it in a non-threatening manner

- Emphasize responsibility

- Read the label of the bottle with them, so they understand the key ingredients to emphasize the dangers of the medication and why the specific dose is used for safety reasons

NIDA reminds parents: "*Despite the concern and widespread abuse DXM products are legal and remain unrestricted, which is why education about these OTCs has to be encouraged at both home and school. These products should be kept away from children and also included in any discussions about addiction. Remember that DXM products are inexpensive and your Internet savvy child knows how to obtain the information they need to purchase it. It just takes a credit or debit card*".

OTC Abuse Goes Beyond DXM:

Over the past decade OTC abuse has taken a very dark turn away from only products sold openly in the pharmacy, and towards products that the user can get that supply a more dangerous effect.

A variety of weight loss supplements are often aimed at women. This group is frequently focused on body image, weight, competition, and self esteem issues. They often wind up abusing OTC diet pills and even herbs trying to lose weight in time for the Prom or the beach, but either they regain the weight or become anorexic. The ingredients are often unknown and as OTCs they are not well regulated.

Inhalants:

The use of inhalants to get high is one of the most frightening and dangerous, relatively new practices by adolescents and adults seeking an illicit drug effect. Again, like OTCs they are legal and found almost anywhere. The only good news about inhalants is that according to NIDA and the University of Michigan Monitoring the Future Studies, there has been a decline in their use and a rise in their perceived danger. There are some signs that use may be increasing in younger adolescents, created by the "generational forgetting" since hazard-education had not been emphasized since the 1990's.

One of the key reasons inhalants are used is that they are readily available and often very inexpensive. Add to that there are more sources and new products that produce the effect as word-of-mouth spreads among users.

Most parents today are more or less clueless when it comes to inhalants because they are a diverse group of volatile substances whose chemical vapors when inhaled produce psychoactive (mind-altering) effects. These substances, unlike cocaine for example are only *inhaled* and are not used intranasally or by injection. They are also not usually found in drug stores or in the pharmacy section of a big box store—rather in hardware stores, supermarkets, and even corner grocery stores.

You may remember that a few decades ago there were "glue sniffers" who used a paper bag to try for a "buzz". Today the inhalants that are being abused are ones that people often avoid, wearing masks such as spray paints, glue, nail polish, gasoline, butane, propellants in products like whip cream and cleaning fluids. Because they are kept around the house or in the garage or basement workshop they are easily opened and experimented with by children of all ages. This would include nitrous oxide in whipped cream dispensers and gas cylinders.

Teenagers who are just experimenting (aged 12-13) usually try glue, shoe polish, spray paints, gasoline, and lighter fluid. Older adolescents (aged 16-17) abuse nitrous oxide or whippets. Nitrites are the class of inhalants most commonly abused by adults.

Inhalants are very dangerous and often fatal. When you "inhale" something, the effect goes to the brain almost instantly. Straight inhalation is called "huffing" but they can also be inhaled through a rag, an aerosol spray, a balloon or a plastic bag. Because the high is quick, the time between doses will often accelerate leading to more potential for overdose.

According to NIDA and other agencies the following inhalants are usually those that are abused:

Volatile solvents—liquids that vaporize at room temperature

- Industrial or household products, including paint thinners or removers, degreasers, dry-cleaning fluids, gasoline, and lighter fluid

- Art or office supply solvents, including correction fluids, felt-tip marker fluid, electronic contact cleaners, and glue

Aerosols—sprays that contain propellants and solvents

- Household aerosol propellants in items such as spray paints, hair or deodorant sprays, fabric protector sprays, aerosol computer cleaning products, and vegetable oil sprays

Gases—found in household or commercial products and used as medical anesthetics

- Household or commercial products, including butane lighters and propane tanks, whipped cream aerosols or dispensers (whippets), and refrigerant gases

- Medical anesthetics, such as ether, chloroform, halothane, and nitrous oxide ("laughing gas")

Nitrites—a special class of inhalants that are used primarily as sexual enhancers
- **Organic nitrites** are volatiles that include cyclohexyl, butyl, and amyl nitrites, commonly known as "poppers." **Amyl nitrite** is still used in certain diagnostic medical procedures. When marketed for illicit use, organic nitrites are often sold in small brown bottles labeled as "video head cleaner," "room odorizer," "leather cleaner," or "liquid aroma"

These various products contain a wide range of chemicals such as:

- toluene (spray paints, rubber cement, gasoline)

- chlorinated hydrocarbons (dry-cleaning chemicals, correction fluids)

- hexane (glues, gasoline)

- benzene (gasoline)

- methylene chloride (varnish removers, paint thinners)

- butane (cigarette lighter refills, air fresheners)

Your Brain On Inhalants:

Groups that monitor inhalant use warn of a number of dangers:

"Sniffing highly concentrated amounts of the chemicals in solvents or aerosol sprays can directly induce heart failure and death within minutes of a session of repeated inhalation. This syndrome, known as "sudden sniffing death," can result from a single session of inhalant use by an otherwise healthy young person. Sudden sniffing death is particularly associated with the abuse of butane, propane, and chemicals in aerosols."

Common effects include:

- Slurred speech, lack of coordination, euphoria, and dizziness

- Lightheadedness, hallucinations, and delusions

- Less inhibited and less in control

- Feeling drowsy

- Chronic headaches

Harmful Irreversible Effects

- Hearing loss—spray paints, glues, dewaxers, dry-cleaning chemicals, correction fluids

- Peripheral neuropathies or limb spasms—glues, gasoline, whipped cream dispensers, gas cylinders

- Central nervous system or brain damage—spray paints, glues, dewaxers

- Bone marrow damage—gasoline

Serious but Potentially Reversible Effects

- Liver and kidney damage—correction fluids, dry-cleaning fluids

- Blood oxygen depletion—varnish removers, paint thinners

Inhalants and Sex:

- Nitrites are frequently used to overcome erectile dysfunction or enhance sexual pleasure and performance; safe sexual practices are not followed, increasing risk of STD's, hepatitis, HIV/AIDS and hepatitis

Inhalant Abuse Data

Monitoring the Future Survey:

According to the Monitoring the Future survey, a significant increase in past-month inhalant use was measured among 10thgraders from 2008 to 2009; prevalence of use rose from 2.1 percent to 2.2 percent among that population. Other prevalence measures remained stable. Lifetime use of inhalants was reported by 14.9 percent of 8th-graders, 12.3 percent of 10th-graders, and 9.5 percent of 12th-graders in 2009; 8.1 percent of 8th-graders, 6.1 percent of 10th-graders, and 3.4 percent of 12th-graders reported use in the past year. However, investigators are concerned that perceived risk associated with inhalant use has been in decline for several years, which may leave young people open to renewed interest.

National Survey on Drug Use and Health (NSDUH):

Data from the National Survey on Drug Use and Health show that the primary abusers of most inhalants are adolescents ages 12 to 17; in 2008, 1.1 percent reported using inhalants in the past month. From 2002 to 2008, there were declines in past-month inhalant use among young adults aged 18 to 25 (from 0.5 percent to 0.3 percent). Of the 729,000 persons aged 12 or older who tried inhalants for the first time within the previous year, approximately 67 percent were under age 18 when they first used.

Other Information Sources:

For additional information on inhalants, please refer to NIDA's inhalant-specific Web site: www.inhalants.drugabuse.gov.

For a list of street terms used to refer to inhalants and other drugs, visit www.whitehousedrugpolicy.gov/streetterms/default.asp.

Club Drugs/MDMA

TV crime show fans will often hear of "club drugs" as part of the plot of a gruesome plotline. Most likely called MDMA, the one most frequently used is also known as Ecstasy. The plot usually involves teens or young people at a wild college party, or clean cut twenty-somethings at a bar or rock concert passing out a number of pills that inevitably leads to some sort of accidental death, date rape or assault. Use of these and other drugs called "club drugs" as a group, have become more widespread over the past three decades and have been easy to obtain.

There are several different drugs used in the club scene, but MDMA is the most abused. With a nickname like 'Ecstasy', the perception of it may not be dangerous as much as something else, for example a safe, stimulant drug. As a synthetic and psychoactive drug MDMA (3,4-methylenedioxymethamphetamine) is actually chemically similar to the stimulants like methamphetamine. Since it produces a sense of more energy, euphoria, emotional warmth—or sexual feelings and a loss of time passing, often the user does not recognize what is going on such as being sexually assaulted.

Who uses club drugs?

MDMA is taken orally, usually as a capsule or tablet and usually by a middle and upper class group with the ability to buy it. According to NIDA,

> ...more recently, the profile of the typical MDMA user has changed, with the drug now affecting a broader range of ethnic groups. MDMA is also popular among urban gay males—some report using MDMA as part of a multiple-drug experience that includes marijuana, cocaine, methamphetamine, ketamine, sildenafil (Viagra), and other legal and illegal substances.

There are two major drugs that are generally associated with MDMA and sometimes called "club drugs". They are known as GHB and Rohypnol:

GHB and **Rohypnol** (also known as "roofies") are available in odorless, colorless, and tasteless forms that are too often used with alcohol and other beverages. GHB and Rohypnol are used to attain a "downed out state" similar to CNS drugs. Both drugs have been used to commit sexual assaults (mentioned above as "date rape," "drug rape," "acquaintance rape," or "drug-assisted" assault) due to their ability to sedate and incapacitate unsuspecting victims, preventing them from resisting sexual assault.

Ketamine, a third drug is a dissociative anesthetic, mostly used in veterinary practice and is usually snorted or injected intramuscularly. Human use is very dangerous. PCP and DXM plus Ketamine create disassociative effects.

Gamma hydroxybutyrate (GHB) is a central nervous system (CNS) depressant that was approved by the Food and Drug Administration (FDA) in 2002 for use in the treatment of narcolepsy (a sleep disorder). This approval came with severe restrictions, including its use only for the treatment of narcolepsy.

- GHB acts in the brain on the GABA(B) receptors and at specific GHB binding sites

- At high doses, GHB's sedative effects may result in SEIZURES sleep, coma, or death

- Users like this drug. It causes disinhibition and increased social ability

- GHB is usually ingested orally, either in liquid or powder form

Side effects associated with GHB may include nausea, vomiting, delusions, depression, vertigo, hallucinations, seizures, respiratory distress, loss of consciousness, slowed heart rate, lowered blood pressure, amnesia, and coma. GHB can become addictive with sustained use.

Rohypnol (flunitrazepam) appeared in the early 1990s. A benzodiazepine (chemically similar to sedative-hypnotic drugs such as Valium or Xanax), but it is not approved for medical use in this country, and its importation is banned.

Rohypnol is typically taken orally in pill form.

Recent reports, however, have shown that Rohypnol is being ground up and snorted; Rohypnol, like other benzodiazepines, acts at the GABA(A) receptor.

Warning: All of these drugs are potentially fatal when used with alcohol or other drugs.

Getting Off Club Drugs:

Club drug use and stopping often means a trip to the emergency room. Users build dependency rapidly and more research is needed to develop any sort of unique recovery program beyond others mentioned in this book. Another problem is that very few ER's actually do see club drug OD's and are not prepared to offer any specific type of treatment. In general, the usual detox program and medical monitoring for any other benzodiazepine is used.

Patients with a ketamine overdose are managed through supportive care for acute symptoms, with special attention to cardiac and respiratory functions.

Club Drug Abuse Data: Monitoring the Future (MTF) Survey

MTF has reported consistently low levels of abuse of these club drugs since they were added to the survey. For GHB and ketamine, this occurred in 2000; for Rohypnol, 1996. According to results of the 2009 MTF survey, 0.7 percent of 8th-grade and 1.1 percent of 12th-grade students reported past-year use of GHB, a statistically significant decrease from peak-year use of 1.2 percent in 2000 for 8th-graders and 2.0 percent for 12th-graders in 2004. GHB use among 10th-grade students was reported at 1.0 percent, an increase from 2008 (0.5 percent), and statistically unchanged from peak use of 1.4 percent in 2002 and 2003.

Past-year use of ketamine was reported by 1.0 percent of 8th-graders, 1.3 percent of 10th-graders, and 1.7 percent of 12th-graders in 2009. These percentages also represent significant decreases from peak years: 2000 for 8th-graders (at 1.6 percent) and 2002 for 10th- and 12th-graders (at 2.2 and 2.6 percent, respectively). For Rohypnol, 0.4 percent of 8th- and 10th-graders, and 1.0 percent of 12th-graders reported past-year use, also down from peak use in 1996 for 8th-graders (1.0 percent), 1997 for 10th-graders (1.3 percent), and 2002 and 2004 for 12th-graders (1.6 percent).

Other Information Sources

For more information about club drugs, visit www.clubdrugs.gov, www.teens.drugabuse.gov, and www.backtoschool.drugabuse.gov; or call NIDA at 877-643-2644. For street terms searchable by drug name, street term, cost and quantities, drug trade, and drug use, visit http://www.whitehousedrugpolicy.gov/streetterms/default.asp.

Heroin:

Heroin is a drug that has caused death and destruction for centuries in the form of opium. Kingdoms have been destroyed over the Asian poppy plant that is the major source of the morphine from the poppy plant used to create heroin. Historically, most of the world's opium has been grown in the infamous *Golden Triangle of Southeast Asia*.

According to the United Nations over the last decade, opium production in the Golden Triangle has declined by over 87 percent while rates in Southwest Asia have increased considerably.

In 2007, Afghanistan supplied 93% of the world's opium. As supply and demand grew, in the late 1990's, Latin America became the most significant distribution pipeline for heroin to the United States. (Mexican heroin was sold on the West Coast while Colombian heroin went to the East Coast)

According to the U.S. Office of National Drug Control,

> "With long-established trafficking and distribution networks and exclusive markets for black tar, brown powder and white heroin, Mexico and Colombia's hold on the U.S. heroin market seems to be secure but cross-regional trafficking is gaining in importance. According to UN reports, there are indications that a small but increasing proportion of opiates from Afghanistan are being trafficked to North America, either via eastern and western Africa, or via Europe."

Abusing Heroin:

The classic image of the heroin user is a degraded, sickly looking person "shooting up" (injecting), snorting, sniffing, or smoking heroin. These methods have the same effect as many other drugs taken this way because the route to the brain is quick if not immediate. These are also the ways that build addiction quickest. When the brain senses the heroin it converts it to morphine where it binds to the "opioid receptors" which are located throughout the brain. These receptors are dedicated to help sense pain and block it or deliver a sense of feeling well.

Opioid receptors are in the brain stem and are vital to simply living such as breathing (respiration), blood pressure, and arousal. Heroin overdoses frequently involve a suppression of respiration.

Why Would Someone Use Heroin & What Will It Do

There are even fewer reasons to use heroin than any other illegal drug, but one really important reason **not** to use is that heroin is highly addictive—added to a high potential for deadly overdose. After shooting heroin—in a vein—the user gets a rush or sense of euphoria accompanied by dry mouth, a warm flushing of the skin, loss of cognitive skills, heaviness of the extremities, and clouded mental functioning.

Next the user begins to nod out, slipping in and out of consciousness "on the nod". Only injecting the drug gives the user the rush but the effects are the same. Many still have severe and permanent damage as a result.

Heroin users that continue to abuse the drug will find that they feel the heroin effect of addiction start to take control of them. Once a user comes down off the high, the desire to obtain more of the drug grows in the form of an obsession or craving. With this obsession also comes a higher tolerance for the drug, meaning more is needed to experience the same heroin effects and high.

If and when a person comes down off heroin, he/she will experience a painful period from detoxing off of the heroin effects. Withdrawal symptoms can include diarrhea, convulsions, vomiting, and uncontrollable body movements. These heroin effects are quite possibly some of the most uncomfortable; however, they will only last for a few days and can be effectively treated with a medical detox and drug treatment.

Heroin And Your Health?

Heroin abuse is associated with serious health conditions including:

- fatal overdose

- spontaneous abortion

- infectious diseases, including HIV/AIDS and hepatitis

- collapsed veins

- infection of the heart lining and valves

- abscesses

- liver or kidney disease

- pulmonary complications

Heroin bought on the street may contain toxic contaminants or additives that can clog blood vessels leading to the lungs, liver, kidneys, or brain, causing permanent damage to vital organs.

WARNING! Chronic use of heroin leads to physical dependence, if user reduces or stops use of the drug abruptly, he or she may experience severe symptoms of withdrawal.

These symptoms—which can begin as early as a few hours after the last drug administration and can:

- include restlessness

- muscle and bone pain

- insomnia

- diarrhea

- vomiting

- cold flashes with goose bumps ("cold turkey")

- kicking movements ("kicking the habit")

- severe craving for the drug during withdrawal

Major withdrawal symptoms peak between 48 and 72 hours after the last dose of the drug and typically subside after about 1 week.

- Some individuals, however, may show persistent withdrawal symptoms for months. Although heroin withdrawal is considered less dangerous than alcohol or barbiturate withdrawal, sudden withdrawal by heavily dependent users who are in poor health is occasionally fatal

- In addition, heroin craving can persist years after drug cessation, particularly upon exposure to triggers such as stress or people, places, and things associated with drug use

- Heroin abuse during pregnancy, together with related factors like poor nutrition and inadequate prenatal care, has been associated with adverse consequences including low birth weight and addicted infants

Treatments:

Heroin treatment includes the usual methods employed such as detoxification, therapy and specific medications that are effective. There are many effective behavioral treatments available for heroin addiction—usually in combination with medication. Examples are individual or group counseling; contingency management, which uses a voucher-based system where patients earn "points" based on negative drug tests—these points can be exchanged for items that encourage healthy living; and cognitive-behavioral therapy.

Medications to help prevent relapse, also called OPM (opiate maintenance therapy) include the following:

Methadone has been used for more than 30 years to treat heroin addiction. It is a synthetic opiate medication that binds to the same receptors as heroin; but when taken orally, it has a gradual onset of action and sustained effects, reducing the desire for other opioid drugs while preventing withdrawal. While this is controversial many point out that this reduces crime and the trade off is a better choice.

Buprenorphine is also a synthetic opioid that is being used for heroin and opioid addiction. It is also used in treatment of withdrawal. Known as a partial agonist, it does not have the full blocking effect on opiate receptors thus Buprenorphine is less reinforcing and unlikely to cause addiction. Rarely does it cause respiratory compromise unless combined with another drug like a CNS depressant like a benzodiazepine. It can be prescribed in a physician's office as an injection, wearable patch, pills or a sublingual patch. It is considered safer than methadone causing less respiratory compromise.

Naltrexone is a long-acting opioid blocker that can be part of a relapse prevention program and approved in use of an alcohol relapse program although it has not been as successful as other agonist blockers. It also is a deterrent for opiate abuse. This medication cannot be used until detoxification is complete to avoid strong withdrawal symptoms. It is administered orally or injected.

Naloxone is a short acting opioid receptor blocker that works by binding to the opiate receptors and blocking opiates from binding to receptors.

Suboxone is a sublingual narcotic medication also used for the treatment of opioid dependence but must be carefully supervised by a physician. It is, like the other drugs, available only by prescription, and must be taken under a doctor's care as prescribed. It is a combination of buprenorphine and naloxone. It prevents the effects of bupenorphine if injected. It is available as a patch or film.

Heroin Abuse Data

Monitoring the Future Survey

According to the Monitoring the Future survey, there was little change between 2008 and 2009 in the proportion of 8th- and 12thgrade students reporting lifetime, past-year, and past-month use of heroin. There also were no significant changes in past-year and past-month use among 10th-graders; however, lifetime use increased significantly among this age group, from 1.2 percent to 1.5 percent. Survey measures indicate that injection use rose significantly among this population at the same time.

National Survey on Drug Use and Health (NSDUH)

According to the 2008 National Survey on Drug Use and Health, the number of current (past-month) heroin users aged 12 or older in the United States increased from 153,000 in 2007 to 213,000 in 2008. There were 114,000 first-time users of heroin aged 12 or older in 2008.

Other Information Sources

For additional information on heroin, please refer to the following sources on NIDA's Web site, www.drugabuse.gov:

Sources: Heroin Abuse—Research Report Series

Various issues of NIDA Notes (search by "heroin" or "opiates") For a list of street terms used to refer to heroin and other drugs, visit www.whitehousedrugpolicy.gov/streetterms/default.asp.

Hallucinogens

If there is any single abused substance that has drawn as much media attention as drugs like crack or pot, it is LSD, a member of a class of synthetic (LSD) and natural drugs (Peyote, mushrooms) called hallucinogenics. They are championed as substances with the ability to cause "changes in a person's perception of reality" but not in the same manner as a CNS depressant or stimulant. Many of these drugs are often used in exotic religious ceremonies and users claim to experience "hallucinations" and report seeing images, sounds and visions that seem very real but aren't.

Hallucinogenic drugs have developed this controversial nature because there is a segment of users who actually believe that by opening their "inner consciousness" they can achieve a more "enlightened state of being."

The popularity of these drugs may be changing. According to the 2010 Monitoring The Future Study: *"For some years, LSD was the most widely used drug within the larger class of hallucinogens. This is no longer true, due to sharp decreases in its use combined with an increasing use of psilocybin.*

"Annual prevalence of LSD use among 12th graders has been below 10% since MTF began. Use declined some for the first 10 years among 12th graders, likely continuing a decline that had begun before 1975. Use was fairly level in the latter half of the 1980s but, as was true for a number of other drugs, rose in all three grades between 1991 and 1996. Since 1996, use has declined in all three grades, with particularly sharp declines between 2001 and 2003; since then use has remained at historically low levels, though there has been a very slight increase in the past few years."

Almost all of these drugs are alkaloids and contain nitrogen with chemical structures similar to those of natural neurotransmitters (e.g., acetylcholine-, serotonin-, or catecholamine-like). Feeding these myths is that it is unclear how these drugs work although it is thought they temporarily interfere with neurotransmitter action or by binding to and blocking these receptor sites.

LSD, peyote, and psilocybin cause their effects by initially disrupting the interaction of nerve cells, specifically the neurotransmitter serotonin. Distributed throughout the brain and spinal cord, the serotonin system is involved in the control of behavioral, perceptual, and regulatory systems, including mood, hunger, body temperature, sexual behavior, muscle control, and sensory perception. On the other hand, PCP acts mainly through a type of glutamate receptor in the brain that is important for the perception of pain, responses to the environment, and learning and memory.

Hallucinogens: Profiles

LSD (d-lysergic acid diethylamide) was discovered in 1938 and is made from lysergic acid, which is found in ergot, a fungus that grows on rye and other grains. "**Acid**" as it is known has been made into tablets, capsules, or a liquid to be put into a sugar cube. It is also frequently put into an absorbing pad of paper and sold as a "tab". In the 1960's it was very popular on college campuses and often even "branded" by the underground labs making them. Users, especially at rock concert and communal activities like "be-ins" went on "trips" lasting about 10-12 hours unless they were overwhelmed by the psychoactive experience and ended up in an ER.

Peyote is a small, spineless cactus in which the principal active ingredient is mescaline. Natives in northern Mexico and the southwestern United States have used this plant as a part of religious ceremonies. Mescaline can also be produced through chemical synthesis. The top of the peyote cactus, also referred to as the crown, consists of disc-shaped buttons that are cut from the roots and dried. These buttons are generally chewed or soaked in water to produce an intoxicating liquid. The hallucinogenic dose of mescaline is about 0.3 to 0.5 grams, and its effects last about 12 hours. Because the extract is so bitter, some individuals prefer to prepare a tea by boiling the cacti for several hours

Psilocybin (4-phosphoryloxy-N,N-dimethyltryptamine) is obtained from certain types of mushrooms that are indigenous to tropical and subtropical regions of South America, Mexico, and the United States. These mushrooms typically contain less than 0.5 percent psilocybin plus trace amounts of psilocin, another hallucinogenic substance. The active compounds in psilocybin-containing "magic" mushrooms have LSD-like properties and produce alterations of autonomic function, motor reflexes, behavior, and perception.

The psychological consequences of psilocybin use include hallucinations, an altered perception of time, and an inability to discern fantasy from reality. Panic reactions and psychosis also may occur.

Mushrooms containing psilocybin are available fresh or dried and are typically taken orally. The effects of psilocybin, which appear within 20 minutes of ingestion, last approximately 6 hours.

PCP (phencyclidine) was developed in the 1950's as an intravenous anesthetic. Its use has since been discontinued due to serious adverse effects. A white crystalline powder that is readily soluble in water or alcohol, it has a distinctive bitter chemical taste. PCP can be mixed easily with dyes and is often sold on the illicit drug market in a variety of tablet, capsule, and colored powder forms that are normally snorted, smoked, or orally ingested. For smoking, PCP is often applied to a leafy material such as mint, parsley, oregano, or marijuana. Depending upon how much and by what route PCP is taken, its effects can last approximately 4–6 hours.

The use of PCP as an approved anesthetic in humans was discontinued in 1965 because patients often became agitated, delusional, and irrational while recovering from its anesthetic effects. PCP is a "dissociative drug," meaning that it distorts perceptions of sight and sound and produces feelings of detachment (dissociation) from the environment and self. First introduced as a street drug in the 1960s, PCP (aka Angel Dust) quickly gained a reputation as a drug that could cause bad reactions and was not worth the risk.

Some abusers continue to use PCP due to the feelings of strength, power, and invulnerability, as well as a numbing effect on the mind that PCP can induce. Among the adverse psychological effects reported are symptoms that mimic schizophrenia, such as delusions, hallucinations, paranoia, disordered thinking, and a sensation of distance from one's environment and violent temper.

Treatment Options

Treatment for alkaloid hallucinogen (such as psilocybin) intoxication—which is mostly symptomatic—is often sought as a result of bad "trips," during which a patient may, for example, hurt him- or herself. Treatment is usually supportive: provision of a quiet room with little sensory stimulation. Occasionally, benzodiazepines are used to control extreme agitation or seizures.

Hallucinogen Data:

According to the National Survey on Drug Use and Health (NSDUH) there were approximately 1.1 million persons aged 12 or older in 2007 who reported using hallucinogens for the first time within the past 12 months.

Monitoring the Future Survey: LSD

There were no significant changes in LSD use from 2007 to 2008 for most prevalence periods among the 8th-, 10th-, and 12th-graders surveyed; however, there was a significant increase in past-month use of LSD among 12th-graders. Perceived risk of harm from taking LSD regularly decreased among 12th-graders (from 67.3 percent in 2007 to 63.6 percent in 2008). No other changes were significant, but longer term trends indicate a steady decline in perceived harmfulness of LSD in all three grades. Such changes in attitude could signal a subsequent increase in use, an outcome that would be of great concern after the large decreases seen since the mid-1990s, when LSD use peaked among youth.

National Survey on Drug Use and Health

In 2007, more than 22.7 million persons aged 12 or older reported they had used LSD in their lifetime (9.1 percent); however, fewer than 620,000 had used the drug in the past year. There was no change between 2006 and 2007 in the number of past-year initiates of LSD.

Peyote and Psilocybin and PCP

It is difficult to gauge the extent of use of these hallucinogens because most data sources that quantify drug use exclude these drugs. The Monitoring the Future survey reported in 2008 that 7.8 percent of high school seniors had used hallucinogens other than LSD—a group that includes peyote, psilocybin, and others—at least once in their lifetime. Past-year use was reported to be 5.0 percent.

Monitoring the Future Survey

In 2008, 1.8 percent of high school seniors reported lifetime use of PCP; past-year use was reported by 1.1 percent of seniors; and past-month use was reported by 0.6 percent. Data on PCP use by 8th- and 10th-graders are not available.

National Survey on Drug Use and Health

In 2007, 6.1 million persons aged 12 or older reported that they had used PCP in their lifetime (2.5 percent), although only 137,000 persons in the same age group reported use in the past year—this represents a decrease from 187,000 persons in 2006.

Other Information Sources

- For more information on hallucinogens and club drugs, please visit www.clubdrugs.gov and www.teens.drugabuse. gov.

- For street terms searchable by drug name, street term, cost and quantities, drug trade, and drug use, visit www. whitehousedrugpolicy.gov/streetterms/default.asp

- For more information on the effects of hallucinogenic drugs, see NIDA's Research Report on Hallucinogens and Dissociative Drugs at www.nida.nih.gov/ResearchReports/ hallucinogens/ hallucinogens.html.

Anabolic Steroids

Anabolic-androgenic steroids (AAS) have grabbed the headlines over the past decade as professional athletes in virtually every sport have admitted to using them for "performance enhancement." "Anabolic" refers to muscle-building, and "androgenic" refers to increased male sexual characteristics. "Steroids" refers to the class of drugs.

These are very dangerous drugs and younger athletes in high school have used them with fatal results. They are also used by young teen males to "look better and buffed". The problem is that the use of AAS by professionals have appeared to produce extraordinary results from Olympic Gold Medals to baseball home run records creating role models for adolescents. This has lead to widespread drug testing programs in a variety of sports, but by targeting AAS drugs that improve performance, some sports have ignored other drugs like marijuana.

It's very important for a parent to be vigilant for the signs of steroid abuse and understand what they actually can do to anyone of any age. The key facts about AAS are:

- They are synthetically produced variants of the naturally occurring male sex hormone testosterone

- These drugs can be legally prescribed to treat conditions resulting from steroid hormone deficiency, such as delayed puberty, as well as diseases that result in loss of lean muscle mass, such as cancer and AIDS

- AAS are taken orally or injected, typically in cycles, rather than continuously. "Cycling" refers to a pattern of use in which steroids are taken for periods of weeks or months, after which use is stopped for a period of time and then restarted

- In addition, users often combine several different types of steroids in an attempt to maximize their effectiveness, a practice referred to as "stacking"

- Pyramiding - starting with a low dose and building up to a higher dose

AAS and The Mind

The immediate effects of AAS in the brain are mediated by their binding to androgen (male sex hormone) and estrogen (female sex hormone) receptors on the surface of a cell. This AAS–receptor complex can then shuttle into the cell nucleus to influence patterns of gene expression. Because of this, the acute effects of AAS in the brain are substantially different from those of other drugs of abuse. The most important difference is that AAS are not euphorigenic, meaning they do not trigger rapid increases in the neurotransmitter dopamine, which is responsible for the "high" that often drives substance abuse behaviors.

AAS and Mental Health

Preclinical, clinical, and anecdotal reports suggest that steroids may contribute to psychiatric dysfunction. Research shows that abuse of anabolic steroids may lead to aggression and other adverse effects. For example, although many users report feeling good about themselves while on anabolic steroids, extreme mood swings can also occur, including manic-like symptoms that could lead to violence.

Addictive Potential:

Animal studies have shown that AAS are reinforcing—that is, animals will self-administer AAS when given the opportunity, just as they do with other addictive drugs. This property is more difficult to demonstrate in humans, but the potential for AAS abusers to become addicted is consistent with their continued abuse despite physical problems and negative effects on social relations. The reality is that the "addictive potential" is really the esthetic effect that the drug has on people—they like the way they look when using this drug.

Withdrawal symptoms are likely when you stop taking AAS including:

- mood swings

- fatigue

- restlessness

- loss of appetite

- insomnia

- reduced sex drive

- depression leading to suicide

- "ROID" RAGE

Steroid abuse—often permanent health effects:

- For *men*—shrinking of the testicles, reduced sperm count, infertility, baldness, development of breasts (gynecomastia), increased risk for prostate cancer, mood swings, acne, difficulty urinating, decreased sperm count, weight gain.

- For *women*—growth of facial hair, male-pattern baldness, changes in or cessation of the menstrual cycle, enlargement of the clitoris, deepened voice, reduced breast size, increased urination, disrupted menstrual cycles, swelling feet.

- For *adolescents*—stunted growth due to premature skeletal maturation and accelerated puberty changes; risk of not reaching expected height if AAS is taken before the typical adolescent growth spurt

- By injecting AAS you run the added risk of contracting or transmitting HIV/AIDS or hepatitis, which causes serious damage to the liver

AAS Data:

Monitoring the Future Survey

Monitoring the Future is an annual survey used to assess drug use among the Nation's 8th-, 10th-, and 12th-grade students. While steroid use remained stable among all grades from 2007 to 2008, there has been a significant reduction since 2001 for nearly all prevalence periods (i.e., lifetime, past-year and past-month use) among all grades surveyed. The exception was past-month use among 12th-graders, which has remained stable. Males consistently report higher rates of use than females: for example, in 2008, 2.5 percent of 12th-grade males, versus 0.6 percent of 12th-grade females, reported past-year use.

Other Information Sources

For a list of street terms used to refer to steroids and other drugs, visit www.whitehousedrugpolicy.gov/streetterms/default.asp

Tobacco:

This book provides information and strategies to protect families from the dangers of addiction and drug abuse of all the myriad classes of drugs. The solutions and information will help families reduce the potential for harm and prevent damage through education and vigilance where children and adolescents are concerned. One substance that is found everywhere is or can be the most difficult challenge to halt—tobacco use.

It would be virtually impossible for anyone of any age to not know that eventually cigarette use will kill you. There are literally thousands of reputable studies that demonstrate all the organ damage smoking causes and the tobacco companies even post a warning on the packages. How many companies tell you before you use their product that it is lethal, but it is easier to purchase than alcohol, which is age restricted. The answer is none, because the tobacco companies are required by law to do this—but unfortunately they build the costs into the price of the cigarettes.

Some Tobacco Facts:

Anyone who is thinking about "looking cool" smoking a cigarette, cigar or chewing tobacco should keep some of these facts in mind:

- Smoking is the fastest route of effect of any drug—whether it's marijuana or crack. Cigarettes work the same way. This fact and the addictive ability of nicotine to keep a smoker going back for more and more makes it dangerous—especially to a developing adolescent brain

- Nearly a quarter of high school students in the U.S. smoke cigarettes

- Another 8% use smokeless tobacco

- Smoking has many health risks for everyone. However, the younger you are when you start smoking, the more problems it can cause

- Health risks can include emphysema, hypertension, and a variety of cancers along with cardiovascular disease

- Nicotine is one of the most heavily used addictive drugs and the leading preventable cause of disease, disability, and death

- The tar in cigarettes increases a smoker's risk of lung cancer, emphysema, and bronchial disorders

- People who start smoking before the age of 21 have the hardest time quitting

- About 30% of youth smokers will continue smoking and die early from a smoking-related disease

- Teen smokers are more likely to use alcohol and illegal drugs

- Second-hand smoke can lead to cancer in teens

- They are more likely to have panic attacks, anxiety disorders, and depression

- U.S. Cigarette smoking accounts for 90% of lung cancer cases in the U.S.

- About 38,000 deaths per year can be attributed to secondhand smoke

- Cigarettes and chewing tobacco are illegal substances in most U.S. states for those under 18; a handful of states have raised the age to 19

Despite all these facts, anti-smoking campaigns for children, adolescents and adults abound. They can be funny or gruesome and they have worked in some ways but obviously from the information above, not well enough. There has been a reasonably steady decline in use and an upswing in disapproval—especially among older teens who may be responding to the media blitzes.

Availability has been mentioned throughout this book as a factor in use leading to abuse and addiction. In the early 1990's 8th grade students reported that getting cigarettes was relatively easy, but that has now dropped significantly. Still, the conundrum that we face in a world of toxins, drug abuse and adolescent addiction is how to prevent tobacco use when adolescents in large numbers can still obtain it easier than most drugs, except perhaps OTCs.

However, it is possible to overcome adolescent and childhood smoking and even to defeat it as an adult. First, parents and other adults who work with children can help by warning them of the risks of smoking. They can also set a good example by not smoking themselves. Next, parents should understand why teens would use tobacco in the face of graphic evidence.

One answer is simple—they are teenagers who like to try different things and be cool. If its "forbidden" it's even more attractive. Smoking, they think draws attention as a "bad-ass". Worse, since smoking is banned in many places, they end up in a single designated smoking spot reinforcing each other. Another surprising fact; they tried their first cigarette in sixth or seventh grade

Most important of all, is that for young children and teens, peer pressure plays a large role in their lives and this is yet another reason why you must remain as vigilant as you would if you suspect marijuana use. This includes considering keeping close tabs on their rooms or noticing some of these signals:

- They often do not perform well in school

- They feel like they are not a part of the school

- They become isolated from other students

- They can't perform as well at sports events

- They feel like they have little hope of going to college

- They feel like they need a job to support their smoking habit

- They are reported to school officials for skipping classes

- They start using other illegal substances

- They begin experimenting with alcohol and other drugs

- They experience pressure from home and school and use tobacco as a form of relief

- Teen smokers enjoy trying to hide their smoking

- Smokeless forms of tobacco are still in use but since 2004 it has diminished. It is almost exclusively male.

How Can You Stop Teen Smoking:

The answer is clear: If you can prevent your child from stopping or not starting before the ages of 18-21, they are far less likely to become a smoker. Additionally, you have to stop or not smoke at all. This is not the same as "you did drugs in the 1960's". You have to be committed to it for the sake of the health of your children.

We know that cigarettes are deadly and nicotine is a drug that is at the top of the "hard to beat" list. The message to your children has to be positive and health related and you have to lead by example. Smoking cessation programs do work in some cases.

Herbal Highs & Synthetic Marijuana:

There are three different herbs or leaves that are used in Central America and are also as "fake marijuana" that are sold on the Internet and on the street. While seemingly innocent and used by anyone looking for a "buzz" they have been closely monitored by the US Drug Enforcement Agency (DEA). They may not be as innocent as many think.

The "fake weed" is developed as an alteration of THC molecule and they, in turn affect the cannabinoid receptors. Of these drugs are found in head shops sold as incense under the names K-2 or Spice, Black Mamba or Gainesville Green.

The DEA has now cracked down. According to a report from the DEA:

> *The United States Drug Enforcement Administration (DEA) is using its emergency scheduling authority to temporarily control five chemicals (JWH-018, JWH-073, JWH-200, CP-47,497, and cannabicyclohexanol) used to make "fake pot" products. Except as authorized by law, this action will make possessing and selling these chemicals or the products that contain them illegal in the U.S. for at least one year while the DEA and the United States Department of Health and Human Services (DHHS) further study whether these chemicals and products should be permanently controlled.*

Over the past year, smokable herbal blends marketed as being "legal" and providing a marijuana-like high, have become increasingly popular, particularly among teens and young adults. These products consist of plant material that has been coated with research chemicals that mimic THC, the active ingredient in marijuana, and are sold at a variety of retail outlets, in head shops and over the Internet. These chemicals, however, have not been approved by the FDA for human consumption and there is no oversight of the manufacturing process. Brands such as "Spice," "K2," "Blaze," and "Red X Dawn" are labeled as incense to mask their intended purpose.

Since 2009, DEA has received an increasing number of reports from poison centers, hospitals and law enforcement regarding these products. Fifteen states have already taken action to control one or more of these chemicals. The Comprehensive Crime Control Act of 1984 amends the Controlled Substances Act (CSA) to allow the DEA Administrator to emergency schedule an abused, harmful, non-medical substance in order to avoid an imminent public health crisis while the formal rule-making procedures described in the CSA are being conducted.

Below are descriptions of the most popular and dangerous "faux pot" products that are widely distributed.

Salvia (*Salvia divinorum*) is an herb common to southern Mexico and Central and South America. The main active ingredient in Salvia, salvinorin A, is a potent activator of kappa opioid receptors in the brain. These receptors differ from those activated by the more commonly known opioids, such as heroin and morphine.

Traditionally, *S. divinorum* has been ingested by chewing fresh leaves or by drinking their extracted juices. The dried leaves of *S. divinorum* can also be smoked as a joint, consumed in water pipes, or vaporized and inhaled.

People who abuse salvia generally experience hallucinations or "psychotomimetic" episodes (a transient experience that mimics a psychosis). Subjective effects have been described as intense but short-lived, appearing in less than 1 minute and lasting less than 30 minutes. They include psychedelic-like changes in visual perception, mood and body sensations, emotional swings, feelings of detachment, and importantly, a highly modified perception of external reality and the self, leading to a decreased ability to interact with one's surroundings.

Extent of Use

In 2009, NIDA's Monitoring the Future Survey of 8th, 10th, and 12th graders asked about salvia abuse for the first time—5.7 percent of high school seniors reported past year use (greater than the percent reporting ecstasy use). Although information about this drug is limited, recent salvia-related media reports and Internet traffic suggest the possibility that its abuse is increasing in the US and Europe, likely driven by drug-related videos and information on Internet sites. Because of the nature of the drug's effects—its use may be restricted to individual experimentalists, rather than as a social or party drug.

For more information on the effects of hallucinogenic drugs, see NIDA's Research Report on Hallucinogens and Dissociative Drugs at www.nida.nih.gov/ResearchReports/hallucinogens/hallucinogens.html.

For more information on Salvia divinorum and the Controlled Substances Act, visit http://www.deadiversion.usdoj.gov/drugs_concern/salvia_d.pdf.

For street terms searchable by drug name, street term, cost and quantities, drug trade, and drug use, visit www.whitehousedrugpolicy.gov/streetterms/default.asp.

"Spice" is used to describe a diverse family of herbal mixtures marketed under many names, including K2, fake marijuana, Yucatan Fire, Skunk, Moon Rocks, and others. These products contain dried, shredded plant material and presumably, chemical additives that are responsible for their psychoactive (mind-altering) effects. While Spice products are labeled "not for human consumption" they are marketed to people who are interested in herbal alternatives to marijuana (cannabis).

Some Spice products are sold as "incense" but resemble potpourri rather than popular, more familiar incense products (common forms include short cones or long, thin sticks). Like marijuana, Spice is abused mainly by smoking. Sometimes Spice is mixed with marijuana or is prepared as an herbal infusion for drinking.

Presently, there are no studies on the effects of Spice on human health or behavior. The U.S. Drug Enforcement Administration (DEA) recently banned five synthetic cannabinoids by placing them in Schedule I status under the Controlled Substances Act. A number of states have also instituted bans on Spice and Spice-like products and/or synthetic cannabinoid-containing products, and many others are considering legislation forbidding the sale or possession of Spice.

Other Information Sources

For more information on Spice and Spice-like products, see Understanding the 'Spice' phenomenon, which was produced by the European Monitoring Centre for Drugs and Drug Addiction: http://www.emcdda.europa.eu/publications/thematic-papers/spice.

Khat (pronounced "cot") is a stimulant drug derived from a shrub (Catha edulis) that is native to East Africa and southern Arabia. The khat plant itself is not scheduled under the Controlled Substances Act; however, because one of its chemical constituents, cathinone, is a Schedule I drug, the Federal Government considers its use illegal.

The main psychoactive ingredients in khat are cathine and cathinone, chemicals that are structurally similar to, but less potent than, amphetamine, yet result in similar psychomotor stimulant effects. Chewing khat leaves can induce a state of euphoria and elation as well as feelings of increased alertness and arousal. The user can also experience an increase in blood pressure and heart rate. The effects begin to subside after about 90 minutes to 3 hours, but can last 24 hours. At the end of a khat session, the user may experience a depressive mood, irritability, loss of appetite, and difficulty sleeping.

There are a number of adverse physical effects that have been associated with heavy or long-term use of khat, including tooth decay and periodontal disease; gastrointestinal disorders such as constipation, ulcers, inflammation of the stomach, and increased risk of upper gastrointestinal tumors; and cardiovascular disorders such as irregular heartbeat, decreased blood flow, and myocardial infarction.

It is unclear whether khat causes tolerance, physical dependency, addiction, or withdrawal, but nightmares and slight trembling have been reported several days after ceasing to chew.

It is estimated that as many as 10 million people worldwide chew khat. It is commonly found in the southwestern part of the Arabian Peninsula and in East Africa, where it has been used for centuries as part of an established cultural tradition. In one large study in Yemen, 82 percent of men and 43 percent of women reported at least one lifetime episode of khat use. No reliable estimates of prevalence in the United States exist.

Other Information Sources

For street terms searchable by drug name, street term, cost and quantities, drug trade, and drug use, visit: www.usdoj.gov/dea/concern/k.html

For more information about club drugs, visit www.clubdrugs.gov, www.teens.drugabuse.gov, and www.backtoschool.drugabuse.gov; or call NIDA at 877-643-2644. For street terms searchable by drug name, street term, cost and quantities, drug trade, and drug use, visit http://www.whitehousedrugpolicy.gov/streetterms/default.asp.

SECTION III:
The UF Prevention and Treatment Methods

Addiction: A Family Affair Florida Rehabilitation Center Case Histories

Addiction treatment, especially at the Florida Recovery Center (FRC) uses an individually designed approach for each patient. Conquering drug addiction is never easy and because we are all distinct from our genetics to our behavior patterns, we've developed methods that can be shaped to each person. This might seem an obvious concept but with a drug related illness it's not the same as treating a cold or an infection.

For example many people become dependent on the *same* drugs—marijuana, painkillers, alcohol—but their roads to and from a rehab center are always different. Some may only be a part-time "weed" user while others with a specific DNA pattern (genetic loading) may smoke less and end up addicted. We have treated thousands of patients who have started off as a social drinker and then one day wake up, not knowing what happened after that third drink.

Why one person is more at risk than another is not merely within the properties of the drug itself or in the patient's lifestyle. In this book we've presented pages of information on the biological process of addiction, the nature and history of various drugs of abuse, and statistics that chart the trends of use by various demographic groups, especially adolescents. These numbers tell us one of the most significant factors that draw different people to a common drug. The U.S. has a unique problem; the *demand for drugs* has not diminished across the board, even though some are used more than others.

New versions of dangerous drugs seem to appear regularly (i.e. "freebasing" cocaine changes to smoking crack) driving this demand and creating new groups of drug addicts who might never have become involved.

A clear goal of the book has been to educate both parents and children about the realities of abused drugs and how to prevent their children from getting involved for a number of reasons. In the next few pages we present some typical cases of real patients we have treated as an illustration of the dangers and destruction drugs can cause to everyone in the family. What all these cases share in common are lives devastated but also lives saved.

Here are some of the underlying principles in the FRC program:

Why The FRC Approach Is Unique: The University of Florida and The Florida Recovery Center is a well-known and respected academic institution conducting serious cutting edge research on brain function and addiction. However, we also shape a person's *continuum of care* program using modern principles of recovery that combine pharmacotherapy, psychotherapy, spirituality, clinical advances with classic treatment that reach into people's families and their hearts and souls. We look at what works with each person and adjust it as treatment continues. No one is fitted into a "typical program".

Inpatient Vs. Outpatient: Not every person who has a problem with addiction has to be hospitalized and in many situations an outpatient program is just as effective. A decision to admit someone to an inpatient program is based on a number of considerations; the need for medical stabilization and also detoxification to remove or "separate environmentally" the patient from access to the drug. There may also be medical needs for underlying medical conditions such as infections, hypertension, or malnutrition.

In making the decision regarding the most appropriate level of care in which to place the patient, there are six dimensions of care and three settings; inpatient, outpatient, and residential.

The six dimensions include:

- **Acute Intoxication And Or Withdrawal Potential**: Is detoxification needed and/or the potential for withdrawal to occur?

- **Bio-Medical Complications And Medications:** What, if any, medical conditions or complications exist? For example is there a history of heart disease, diabetes, hepatitis or STDs?

- **Emotional Behavioral Or Cognitive Condition And Complications:** Are there any emotional, behavioral or cognitive conditions and complications such as co-existing psychiatric conditions, including mood disorders, grief and loss, shame and guilt that will influence the treatment plan?

- **Readiness For Change:** Is the patient exhibiting readiness for change? Are they sincerely motivated and how much denial do they have? Do they just want to avoid the consequences of what has happened? How do we get them from that point to really want to change? Most people deny they have the illness—especially the severity of the illness and what it takes to recover.

- **Relapse Continued Use Potential**: Relapse risk and potential to relapse is common and coping strategies have to be designed to understand how deal with the consequences.

- **Recovery Environment:** What is the environment of someone recovering? What will they have to cope with? Where will they live? Who do they live with? Do they have legal or financial problems? All of this is a keystone to development of a truly shaped, successful drug and alcohol recovery program?

Detoxification Approach: The FRC detox program is not similar to any other program. It examines the patient's whole risk (see above) but the emphasis initially is on medical safety and a humane environment. The second goal is to separate the patient from the drug and this might only be carried out in a medical facility and can be a longer process. In many cases elsewhere medication is used and these combinations with an alcoholic, for example, can be lethal. Care is always taken to ensure safety of the patient. Withdrawal methods that work best with each patient are usually specific to the drug being used. Some do not cause as much personal turbulence and in some case such as adolescents, detox can be a shorter period.

Re-Entry Into The Community may be one of the most difficult steps. We put great emphasis on relapse prevention and see that the patient does complete the program's continuum of care. We take the time to create transition programs that can include day or weekend furloughs, commuting to programs, attending group programs, and rebuilding life skills.

Family Involvement It is a critical component of recovery and families must participate since drug abuse affects the entire family. The destruction and dysfunction has to be addressed and resolved.

PJ

PJ, a scrawny teenager, wearing jeans and a "Lil Wayne" t-shirt sat across from me in the "meeting room" a comfortable den-like space where we talked one-on-one to patients who have entered treatment at the Florida Rehab Center (FRC). I'd seen him before, sadly, starting at age nine. It was clear even then that I had to reach deeper and find a path for this young man who was trying very hard to get back to a normal life. Now he was about to be discharged.

Unfortunately for PJ, his road away from drugs was still going to continue to be difficult because he clearly had a combination of a primary psychiatric illness and was a long time drug abuser. While these were two distinct illnesses, they both dramatically affected his behavior like intertwined vines, choking him.

PJ was back at the FRC this time when his parents noted a worsening depression but also discovered evidence of alcohol, marijuana and opiate use both in his room and car. Now his parents were even more concerned (if possible) because they also discovered that he was using drugs intravenously ("shooting up").

The most significant aspect of PJ's current stint in rehab is that he came back on his own. He told me, "I underestimated the importance of not seeing my old friends and became too comfortable with that old group."

We had identified something that was buried deeply, and perhaps driving his drug use and depression was the fact that he was adopted,. This, he learned was something doctors call a "primal wound" but translated to a feeling that he "was not worth keeping" by his biological parents.

PJ was able to overcome these feelings of rejection and pain to begin moving on.

This marked the end of a very sad period for PJ. Our first meeting had been 10 years ago when he was only nine—not even out of elementary school. While not uncommon, drug use at that age was not usually the way children "acted out."

However, as I got deeper into his story, it was clear that he had many risk factors that would lead him to submerge his feelings with drugs. Even now, sitting with him and talking I remembered him clearly at nine years old in treatment for drugs, depression, and anxiety. His depression was severe enough to warrant treatment with antidepressants despite his young age.

The first thing we did when I saw him at nine was to explore his family history in depth, searching for reasons that PJ was suffering and self-destructing. One answer jumped out immediately and was common in many young drug users' histories. PJ was adopted.

PJ's adoptive parents were well off and professionals. His mother was a successful trial lawyer and his father was a real estate developer. According to both of them and PJ, they were attentive to his needs, somewhat indulgent and involved—helping with homework or other needs.

I learned that PJ was adopted out of difficult circumstances and an only child. These were two of many red flags in his life. His biological parents were both alcoholics and depressives who self medicated with opiates. Ultimately PJ's father was incarcerated and the state removed him from the mother and he went to a group home for some normalcy. Then after a year in foster care, his new parents adopted him but in the end he never met his biological mother who ultimately died of an overdose. He had no other family.

This history was very significant. Both adoptive parents were mature 30 something adults when he was adopted and they were told about the depression and alcoholism in his biological parents. They chose to take a chance. His adoptive parents were high functioning professionals who had no history of alcohol, drug-related or psychiatric problems and felt they could overcome the problem with love and attention.

When I saw PJ for the first time at nine, his new family had not given up on him and in fact felt some sense of responsibility. He was successfully treated that first time but it was not too long before we met again.

PJ was treated two more times over the years. The next time was at age 15 for a period of three months as an adolescent inpatient. But a year later he was back for another three month stay. While he struggled in his initial treatment, he was clearly making an effort and he had his family supporting him. PJ was not a bad kid—rather a sick one and I felt that each time we were getting closer to a treatment plan that would work.

At his third treatment event—he was now 15—he was stabilized on antidepressants and became engaged in 12-Step recovery. His denial lessened as his treatment progressed and his depression was adequately managed with a combination of Lexapro and Wellbutrin.

He was soon out of treatment and initially did quite well, going back to school and getting a part-time job. As he became more successful in school and started doing better, he slipped back in with his old friends and their crowd. Within in a month or two he'd justified some "weekend" partying and drinking to be part of the cool group. This was followed a few months later by return to prescription pain meds, available to him from friends or dealers.

PJ was not a voluble or particularly articulate teen but justified his drinking and drug use simply saying: "I want people to think I'm cool."

This thought process—common for teens—really was the underlying rationale that brought him back to FRC the third time. His parent now knew the signs and wanted him to get help before he went on to intravenous use and they participated fully. Unfortunately, a pattern was developing. PJ would finally acknowledge during his second time in treatment that it really was not "cool" to be in rehab. As a result PJ began another effort but following his pattern, at first he succeeded but then:

- After discharge, he quickly became complacent and was not consistent in taking his antidepressants,

- Although initially attending numerous 12-Step meetings, he cut back significantly once he started to get some success,

- He returned to hanging around with his drug-using peers; thinking that he would not use but wanted to be friends with them.

This time he was an adult and had gone through a fourth treatment cycle. During the pre-discharge meeting in the "den", we talked about his responsibilities and potential consequences both physiological and legal. PJ was clearly able to process what he had done well and what he had poorly. This treatment had lasted two months of partial hospitalization with a housing component followed by a third month spent commuting from home. Today he is doing well and has returned to school.

Today he is over three years sober.

What PJ's Story Tells Us:

- Driving PJ's problems were a clear genetic pre-disposition to addiction and psychiatric problems that are often common in adoptions. This is sometimes called the Primal Wound and over the years this was also a target of his treatment.

- P.J. never met his parents and yet had the genetic predisposition to depression, alcohol and drug addiction. Despite being loved by two supportive parents, they could not stop the occurrence of the illness, which may have been transferred to him while his mother was pregnant.

- P.J. clearly had a dual diagnosis and was already being treated for depression and anxiety at the age of nine before he ever started using drugs.

- When he came to treatment, it was very clear that these two independent disorders had to be dealt with and the issues of using medications for a child that young were discussed at length. Drug addiction and a primary psychiatric illness both need to be treated aggressively. It is not that one led to the other, but he had two separate illnesses, both dramatically influencing the other.

- Other lessons from this case include complacency that occurred for this patient as well the importance of the influences of peers, especially with regard to the young people P.J. started hanging around with while thinking he would not return to using.

CT

C.T. came to our treatment center after being transferred from the psychiatric unit. He had failed in an effort to commit suicide and had been was hospitalized after being stabilized at the University of Florida, Shands Teaching Hospital.

The details of CT's suicide attempt left no doubt that he had serious psychiatric problems and was quite sick. C.T. had shot himself in the head while drunk. Amazingly, the bullet did not enter into his brain but somehow only hit his skull. After being stabilized medically, C.T. was "Baker Acted" (a law that provides emergency medical care and also detention for certain patients) and transferred to the psychiatric unit where he was diagnosed with Major Depressive Disorder as well as Alcohol Dependence.

After his stint as an in-patient, CT came into our treatment center initially depressed but expressing a glimmer of hope. Considering that he had tried to shoot himself, he denied any suicidal ideation. Breaking that enormous level of denial would take four months in our treatment program at Florida Recovery Center.

During this time we discovered significant family history. His grandfather suffered from alcohol dependence but there were no signs of trauma or abuse. The fact that he was unmarried weighed heavily on him.

Eventually he was able to do well on a single anti-depressant. His mood and depression lifted and he immersed himself in the recovery process. Like many people who attempt suicide, the opportunity to actually live gave him a greater sense of enthusiasm and threw him into 12-Step recovery. CT's treatment at the Florida Recovery Center included individual therapy, antidepressant regime and 12-Step recovery. He left to live in a half-way house for another year.

Today, four years down road, CT is clean and sober and is truly one of the miracles of treatment and AA. C.T. recently attended our reunion and spoke of his gratitude and his journey. Today he works fulltime as a chef in a nearby city and is even in a fulfilling relationship. He continues on his antidepressant but finds his life and enjoyment of his job to be a major part of his life.

Lessons from this case:

- **There was a biological predisposition of alcoholism.**
Although not present in C.T.'s parents, it skipped a generation as his grandfather suffered from alcoholism. Genetic predisposition is often present, sometimes you have to look back a generation.

- **The synergy of addiction and major depression disorder.**
A common suicide story is that of a patient with a major depression disorder and a co-morbid addiction.

- **Other issues of importance** are that C.T. lived in a halfway house for one year after discharge. He had a continuum of care as he participated in intensive outpatient treatment after discharge for a period of four to five months. Continuum of care is critical as we move the patient from one level of care to another as it keeps them actively involved in the treatment process and monitoring, which he was for one year. He is truly a miracle of recovery.

HM

HM came to our treatment center as a 42 year old male physician sent by a Physician's Health Program. His colleagues were very concerned after HM was seen by a psychiatrist who confirmed their concerns about H.M.'s mental status.

We soon discovered that over several years H.M. had become dependent on opiates (pain meds), benzodiazepines (anti-anxiety) and numerous other substances, mostly sedative in nature. Other drugs that he abused included high doses of psych stimulants to combat the sedative nature of his opiates and sedatives. H.M. also had a history of obsessive compulsive disorder (OCD) and a dependent personality disorder as well.

In short, HM was in real trouble and maintaining his medical license was the very least of his problems. He had also developed a significant cognitive impairment for some time in treatment. His cognitive impairment was so significant that it took a good three to four months for him to "unbake". He was treated for a total of nine months before he began to show some progress.

HM's downfall was the combination of sedative and psychostimulants along with the patient's psychiatric comorbidity (anxiety and depression) combined to make him too impaired to return to practice. Other issues included a family history of alcohol dependence in his grandfather, a very over-protective, over-bearing mother and the lack of any significant relationships in his life.

HM was gay but had no significant other, never married nor did he have any children. He had not had a relationship with another male for many years.

Even after he was detoxified, treated and sober, he would continue to be rather anxious. His OCD was actively treated with pharmacotherapy as well as CBT (Cognitive Behavioral Therapy). H.M. would be monitored in the Physician's Health Program in his state for a period of five years.

Sadly, he would never return to the practice of medicine because of the severity of his cognitive impairment as well as his OCD. He would, however, stay sober and has been sober now for eight years. He continues to be managed pharmacologically and with individual therapy. He is active in AA and is very grateful for his recovery.

Lessons from this case:

The most significant is that HM developed severe cognitive impairment from long-term drug use. His years of abuse of psychostimulants, benzodiazepines, and alcohol created enough damage that he could not recover enough to practice medicine with reasonable skill and safety. This case also illustrates how other psychiatric issues such as OCD can be aggressively managed and treated in addition to the patient's alcohol and drug-related problems. Other issues in this case were the need for long-term treatment as this patient was treated for nine months and needed every day of it.

PA

P.A., a well-known surgeon, was sent to our treatment center after both his wife and mother contacted us. They facilitated the admission and his mother even brought him to the treatment center since she was concerned that one day he might harm a patient.

His wife was equally concerned and terrified because he became very angry when he drank and was verbally abusive. His colleagues were concerned and discussed it but had never intervened.

PA was not cooperative initially and resisted any treatment. Initially, he wanted to leave and it took a visit from his mother and a clear mandate that if he did not complete treatment, he would be reported to the State Board and it would be recommended that he not be allowed to practice and any attempt to do so could possibly harm a patient.

More significantly, he demonstrated serious brain problems. His neuro-cognitive testing showed serious deficits in processing speed and memory. Processing speed was less than the 5th percentile (for the general population). Another factor in PA's case was his strained relationship with his son and daughter, both of whom were older. Surprisingly he actually did not see the connection between his alcoholism and these strained relationships. This would change.

As we learned more of his social and medical history we learned that his father left the home when PA was quite young for another woman. This created significant pain which needed to be addressed in P.A.'s treatment. P.A. was able to begin to resolve his feelings during his first four months at the Florida Recovery Center.

Ultimately his denial would lessen and he would become more emotionally vulnerable especially when discussing the pain of his father's actions in his life. He was able to recognize his anger and saw how when he drank, it worsened. His relationship dramatically improved with his wife, mother and eventually with his two children.

We did discover one really important factor that resulted from his substance abuse. Although his cognitive testing improved, it was still abnormal three months into treatment. His cognitive function would never return to a normal range, which would not allow him to practice surgery until one year after treatment. He stays monitored by the Physician's Health Program in his State, remains drug and alcohol free and eventually did return to practice and is doing well today.

Lessons from this case:

Lessons from this case are numerous but a significant one is the cognitive impairment associated with alcoholism. It took one year for P.A. to return to his level of function that would allow him to practice surgery. Despite the fact that he did not drink for three months and sounded okay, he still had impaired neuro-cognition. This is not always easily noted in conversations.

This physician, although quite successful in his life, clearly had emotional wounds from his father leaving at a young age. This needed to be addressed as part of his treatment. Although we say alcoholism is a disease of the brain, recovery must involve healing of the heart of soul.

It took a family intervention for him to get to treatment and we needed both the carrot and the stick. We needed his mother to tell him that he needed to stay in treatment as well as the mandate if he wanted to return to the practice of medicine, he needed to comply with our recommendations.

His colleague's hesitancy to intervene on him speaks to the conspiracy of silence, not only in medicine but in many areas of life where people are hesitant to express their concerns to someone who suffers from drug addiction and alcoholism. Once again, this is a good example of the need for long-term treatment and close monitoring after treatment.

PB

P.B. was a 17-year-old high school junior when I met him. He was transferred to our Addiction Inpatient Unit from the Child and Adolescent Unit where he was initially hospitalized after being sent from an emergency room.

He was rushed to the hospital by his parents after they found him barely breathing in their bathroom at home. P.B. had been diagnosed with a malignant bone tumor that was found in his leg quite accidently following a soccer game. Originally, P.B. had thought he had injured his leg when the mass was found.

- P.B. was a star high school player locally and was quite a good student. He was well known to his teammates as an easy-going guy who liked to smoke pot. His history would reveal that he had used marijuana since his freshman year, smoking rather regularly which resulted in him going from a straight A to a B-C student; but it was not his pot-smoking that brought him to our treatment center.

- P.B. was found on the bathroom floor because he had overdosed on his pain medicines. P.B. was diagnosed with an inoperative sarcoma of his leg beginning in his junior year. He came to us at the end of his junior year. He was originally exposed to opioid pain medicines because of the nature of his illness.

He had severe and nagging pain from his surgery as well as significant side effects from his chemotherapy. He would require more and more medicine to relieve his pain and it was unknown to his oncologist that he was abusing pain medications but a physician's assistant who was a recovering individual discovered it.

The PA expressed significant concern about P.B.'s use of his pain medications but no one paid much attention when he pointed out his concern in the months prior to P.B.'s respiratory event.

P.B. would come to the Florida Recovery Center and struggle with treatment. He was only 17 and quite devastated from his diagnosis of cancer. He was clinically depressed and knew he had a problem with opiates and found that they not only treated his physical pain but provided great relief from the emotional and physic pain of his dual conditions

We elected to keep P.B. on Suboxone, partial opioid agonist pain medication, to treat his chronic pain and to quiet his cravings for opiates. P.B. struggled and was treated on three different occasions at the Florida Recovery Center: two times in extended residential setting and one time in intensive outpatient.

P.B. struggled for three years, initially with a combination of continued chemotherapy for his cancer, which caused significant physical and emotional discomfort as well as clinical depression and a hesitancy to truly become clean and sober. His maintenance on Suboxone kept him in and around the program while frequent random urine testing caught a couple relapses on marijuana.

There were a few instances in which he took more Suboxone than was prescribed, but he was able to honestly acknowledge this to us.

Critical therapeutic issues surrounding his case was getting this young man to identify and express uncomfortable feelings, not only associated with his diagnosis but associated with his parent's divorce which happened approximately two years before his diagnosis of cancer.

What was critical about P.B.'s case is that he stayed around the program and would acknowledge his slips. We developed a good relationship and he never felt judged for his relapses; this was critical for his success.

Other aspects of this case that are significant are P.B.'s initial abuse and dependence of marijuana as well as his initial exposure to opiates for quite a legitimate reason but then using his medical problems as a vehicle to obtain opiates. People felt sorry for him, as he was a young man with cancer and he was able to use his charming, manipulative ways to get more opiates from his physicians who may have had a hard time seeing a 17-year-old middle class solid student soccer player as a drug addict. This is a common theme as people with legitimate pain problems also may find that they like and enjoy opiates and they use their medical problem as a vehicle to obtain opiates.

Physicians stigmatize addiction and have a hard time understanding that both chronic pain and addiction can co-exist. This case also illustrates the tremendous pain that children feel when the parents get divorced. Finally this case underscores marijuana's impairment on learning as this young man went from an A student to a B-C student in high school.

FL

FL was twenty year old young woman when she came to Florida Recovery Center for the first time. She came to us after failing treatment in an intensive outpatient setting in her hometown on the west coast of Florida.

Her history was that she had been exposed to oxycodone as a junior in high school when her friends told her about the wonderful high obtained by eating Oxyies. When she first tried them she told me she "immediately had a sense of well-being and a sense of energy". Her parents also noted a change in her behavior in her junior year of high school and by her senior year, at age eighteen, they took her to her first counseling sessions to deal with this problem with individual therapy.

FL saw an individual therapist for many months but continued to use during this period. FL was one of three children from a middle class background where her parents were happily married. There were no overwhelming traumas in FL's life and she was a solid A/B student, with normal interests before experiencing opiates during her junior year in high school. Her first treatment was as a senior and involved more individual therapy.

After her parents realized that she was still using drugs they started her in an intensive outpatient program in her hometown on the West coast of Florida. FL remained interested in recovery and as a senior in high school did actually complete an outpatient program for the first time.

FL continued to do well, graduated high school and began community college the following year. She had moved out of her house and had convinced her parents that she was not using drugs. She did have short period of time of abstinence from opiates but never completely stopped participating in the party scene which included drinking and smoking marijuana.

At community college she quickly started hanging around with a group of friends and returned to the use of oral opiates because "they were her favorite buzz." Toward the end of her first year, her mother came for a visit and found some pills in FL's room and confronted her. FL did admit she had returned to the use of opiates and agreed to go back into an intensive outpatient program while she continued in community college.

In reality, FL was really only attending the outpatient program (IOP) to please her mother and father, and had very little interest in recovery. As a result, FL did not do well at IOP and it was recommended that she receive a higher level of care, and she was referred to us at Florida Recovery Center. We quickly determined and it was apparent that she was not just taking opiates orally. Eight months prior to coming to Florida Recovery Center she had begun injecting opiates., introduced to her by her boyfriend. She was too ashamed to admit to her parents the use of IV opiates but had to eventually do so when she was diagnosed with Hepatitis C upon admission into our treatment center. She was devastated by this as she had sworn to only using clean needles and not sharing needles.

FL was full of shame about being an IV drug abuser and it was very difficult to tell her parents about this and the diagnosis of Hepatitis C. Her parents were flabbergasted and did not know what to do. There was much attention and much focus placed on her Hepatitis C and how tragic this was. There seemed to be a greater fear about the consequences of Hepatitis C in both her and her parents then there was from her disease of drug addiction.

Fl was able to acknowledge that once she learned to inject opiates that the high was superior to when she took them orally, therefore she had become attached to this. Also interesting in FL's case was that she was initially seen by a therapist and a psychiatrist while a junior in high school. She lied to everyone about her drug use and was initially diagnosed with a depressive disorder and placed on anti depressants.

Admitting and acknowledging that she wanted to focus more on the depressive symptoms with her therapist and psychiatrist meant she did not want to tell them the truth about her drug use. This led her to being treated with various anti depressants, none of which worked. She came to us as she was taken off anti depressants and her mood and affect were followed closely. To overcome the shame of being an IV drug abuser and getting FL's family involved in treatment she did play well and was able to complete a 90 day treatment program. Fl seemed to be very positive about recovery upon discharge.

Initially, FL attended many meetings and was active in recovery and stable off anti-depressants. At approximately six months sobriety FL and her family became more worried about the Hepatitis C. They went to a liver specialist and it was decided that she would be treated with Interferon anti-viral medication that is used in the treatment of Hepatitis C. She has not consulted an addiction medicine specialist and began Interferon at six months of sobriety. This medicine is associated with significant depressive symptomatology, which can be overwhelming for someone early in recovery. The parent's decision to begin Interferon treatments was made with the thinking that her addiction was a cured problem and that the focus needed to be on treating her Hepatitis, which, at the time, was not an active issue. FL slowly decreased her attendance at meetings, and started to hang around with some of her old friends, who convinced her that it was okay to drink occasionally. FL stopped going to meetings, and began to just drink socially while she was taking the Interferon for her Hepatitis C.

She became somewhat more depressed with the use of Interferon and her drinking increased. She did not want to come back to treatment as she thought she could drink like a normal human begin and her primary problem was opiates.

During this period, her parents did not notice any problems associated with her return to social drinking. FL's drinking escalated and her depression worsened. She went back and saw her original psychiatrist, who once again placed her on numerous and various anti depressants. It would be two years before FL would return to our treatment center and by that time she was on three different psychotropic medications for her depression and had returned to the use of IV opiates and had been using them for one and half years. She was too full of shame to tell her parents about the return to her IV drug use and when they finally found out they insisted that she come back to treatment, but that was two years later.

FL would return to treatment acknowledging that she had returned to the use of IV opiates one and a half years ago and had lied to her therapist and psychiatrist once again about her return to use. Focus was placed on her psychiatric issues and there were numerous medications tried. FL has recently re-entered treatment and has been here now for two months. She has asked to come off her psychotropic medications, which she has been successfully weaned off. She is just starting to get some hope again and she expressed significant shame about her return to usage stating that she did not want to tell her parents and that is why it took almost two years for her to come back into treatment following her relapse.

Her case illustrates numerous points:

1   The increase in prescription drug use on our high school population. FL's first exposure was not because of her pain problem but just to get high. Her friends were well aware of the euphorigenic nature of opiates and FL tried them and immediately liked them.

2   FRC physicians and staff see more and more of the progression of the use of oral opiates to intravenous use. FL would not be considered the classic IV drug abuser. She is now one of many young people that I have seen who had started using orally and have progressed to IV. This was shocking for her family.

3   This case also illustrates the significant change vacillated by IV drug use and its consequences as FL has Hepatitis C even though she claims she always used clean needles.

4   Hepatitis C is common with IV drug abuse and studies show anywhere from 60-90% of people who inject drugs will be positive for Hepatitis C regardless of their report of using clean needles or not sharing them.

5   FL's case also illustrates how her family became complacent about her recovery. It was shortly after her discharge that she thought that she could drink normally because her problem was opiates. She began with exposure to alcohol and before a short period of time was back to using opiates intravenously. This is a very progressive disease and each time that someone returns to use, the consequences seem to get more severe as the disease progresses. Also, significant in this case, is that it took one and a half to two years for FL to come back to treatment after returning to use. People do not always come back to treatment right away and some never make it back.

6   This case also illustrates how addiction is a great masquerade; FL was too ashamed to admit to her therapist and counselor about her injecting drugs. She wanted to talk more about her depressive symptomatology which was easier to discuss. Drug addiction can coexist with psychiatric problems but in this case stemmed from them. Her true problem was not depression

but drug addiction. She was able to fool her therapist on two different occasions. The first therapist and psychiatrist believed her about not using drugs and never tested her when she was a senior in college. Once again the same mistake was made after starting her therapy. This might have indeed been the case but nobody was drug testing her or asking about her return to drug usage.

7   This case illustrates the importance of continued testing as a method for monitoring drug and alcohol addiction. Taking a drug addict's word that they are clean and sober is a big mistake. Not following people with the disease of drug addiction by testing them is like treating somebody with an antihypertensive and not checking their blood pressure, it is just wrong and bad medicine.

RM

RM was a thirty-two year old young male when he first came to our treatment center. He was brought to the center by his parents who were terribly worried about his problematic drinking. He had a long history of alcohol related problems as well as a very significant history of anxiety, which he saw as his primary problem. He had two DUIs and had a charge of disorderly conduct secondary to his drinking. He had no other legal history beyond those situations that were alcohol involved.

RM also had a significant problem with Benzodiazepines; he would take Xanax to relieve his anxiety which he said was overwhelming. He had been diagnosed with generalized anxiety disorder and social phobia in his early twenties. He had been in therapy and psychiatric treatment for many years before he had ever entered treatment for his alcohol related problems. He would acknowledge that alcohol made it easy for him to talk to people and that is why he started drinking in his late teens.

Both he and his parents would report that his drinking did not become problematic or at least apparent, until his mid twenties when he experienced a DUI. RM saw his primary problem as his anxiety disorder and insisted that he only drank and took Xanax to relieve his anxiety. His belief was that if his anxiety could be adequately managed he would not need to drink or take Xanax.

The FRC was RM's third treatment center, as he had left his two previous treatment centers against medical advice as they would not leave him on Benzodiazepines as he requested. Because of RM's tendency to drink and drive, his two DUIs and his legal history we were able to convince his parents to mandate RM's treatment, as once again he wanted to leave if he was not given Benzodiazepines.

This time RM was court ordered to treatment. He stayed in treatment for a period of four months and initially was argumentative and very married to his anxiety disorder. He thought his alcoholism and his Xanax problem secondary to untreated anxiety. We were able to hold on to RM long enough to convince him that although he did suffer with a very real and significant anxiety disorder he also had the disease of alcoholism and drug addiction that needed to be treated along with his anxiety disorder.

We were able to successfully and slowly taper him off his Benzodiazepines and treat him with Lexapro (SSRI which is used to treat depression and anxiety) along with cognitive behavioral therapy. The combination of an SSRI and CBT helped him with his anxiety disorder. We were also able to get him to see how the program of A.A. and spiritual recovery program helped him stay sober, improve his life, and also help with his anxiety disorder and depression.

RM was also able to learn other non pharmacologic coping strategies to deal with his anxiety including meditation and daily exercise. He learned to enjoy biking and jogging and over time was able to see how these dramatically helped his anxiety disorder. Family therapy was also a critically part of RM's treatment.

This case illustrates some critical points:

1   Alcoholism and drug addiction can co-occur with other disorders specifically mood and anxiety disorder.

2   RM had a very real anxiety disorder which needed to be treated. However, his alcoholism and drug addiction were not secondary to his anxiety disorder but alongside it. They both needed to be treated and treating one would not get rid of the other, this is a critical issue that surfaces again and again in this field. Often it is not an issue of this or that treatment but this plus that treatment.

3   RM's case also illustrates the importance of being very careful when treating people with addictive disorder, short acting drugs that have a high addiction liability; Xanax is one of these drugs. Although RM had a very real anxiety disorder, and needed pharmacotherapy it was important to stay away from short acting drugs which are reinforcing, as is the case with Xanax.

4   RM's case also illustrates the importance of treating people with addictive disorders and not dismissing their coexisting problems. RM's anxiety disorder was very real and needed to be addressed but he also needed to be convinced that his alcohol and drug problem was very real. This takes time.

5. His case also illustrates the potential for the legal system and the treatment world to work together. RM was mandated to treatment because of his DUIs and disorderly conduct charges. In his case, mandated treatment allowed us to hold onto him to allow changes to occur in his heart.

TAKE ACTION NOW!

As you see in this book substance abuse and drug addiction have now become America's # 1 health problem and we are at a turning point in the way our country addresses this crisis. It is my hope that this book will serve as a wake-up call to every adult in America.

Tackling drug abuse and addiction will help our children avoid accidents, injuries and a wide range of medical and psychiatric problems as well as unintended pregnancies, criminal involvement and even death. Without drug abuse, our children will perform better academically and adults will succeed professionally. All of us can help cut the chances of acquiring a lifetime of chronic and debilitating illness.

The solution to the broad-based drug abuse wave must include helping the public understand the risks of early introduction of drugs to adolescents as well as the nature of addiction and its origin as a pediatric onset illness.

We must:

- Prevent or delay the onset of substance usage as long as possible through the implementation of effective public healthcare measures and identify teens at risk for substance use through teen screens as we do for other healthcare problems.

- Intervene early when we see a problem to avoid further usage and its consequences and we must be able to provide appropriate treatment for people having a substance-use or co-occurring disorder.

We must also recognize the critical role of parental attitudes towards alcohol and drugs and how this impacts our children as much as the genetics that we pass along to them. The problem is that we have failed to act.

It is time to muster the motivation that will recognize this as a public health problem that it will take a combination of healthcare professionals, parents, policy-makers, educators, media, researchers and the teens themselves to act together.

I maintain the hope that we can accomplish this.

Appendix A: Results from the 2009 National Survey on Drug Use and Health

Introduction

This report presents a first look at results from the 2009 National Survey on Drug Use and Health (NSDUH), an annual survey of the civilian, noninstitutionalized population of the United States aged 12 years old or older. The report presents national estimates of rates of use, numbers of users, and other measures related to illicit drugs, alcohol, and tobacco products. The report focuses on trends between 2008 and 2009 and from 2002 to 2009, as well as differences across population subgroups in 2009. Estimates from NSDUH for States and areas within States will be presented in separate reports. NSDUH estimates related to mental health, which have been included in national findings reports in prior years, are not included in this 2009 report.

Highlights

This report presents the first information from the 2009 National Survey on Drug Use and Health (NSDUH), an annual survey sponsored by the Substance Abuse and Mental Health Services Administration (SAMHSA). The survey is the primary source of information on the use of illicit drugs, alcohol, and tobacco in the civilian, noninstitutionalized population of the United States aged 12 years old or older. The survey interviews approximately 67,500 persons each year. Unless otherwise noted, all comparisons in this report described using terms such as "increased," "decreased," or "more than" are statistically significant at the .05 level.

Illicit Drug Use

- In 2009, an estimated 21.8 million Americans aged 12 or older were current (past month) illicit drug users, meaning they had used an illicit drug during the month prior to the survey interview. This estimate represents 8.7 percent of the population aged 12 or older. Illicit drugs include marijuana/ hashish, cocaine (including crack), heroin, hallucinogens, inhalants, or prescription-type psychotherapeutics used nonmedically.

- The rate of current illicit drug use among persons aged 12 or older in 2009 (8.7 percent) was higher than the rate in 2008 (8.0 percent).

- Marijuana was the most commonly used illicit drug. In 2009, there were 16.7 million past month users. Among persons aged 12 or older, the rate of past month marijuana use and the number of users in 2009 (6.6 percent or 16.7 million) were higher than in 2008 (6.1 percent or 15.2 million) and in 2007 (5.8 percent or 14.4 million).

- In 2009, there were 1.6 million current cocaine users aged 12 or older, comprising 0.7 percent of the population. These estimates were similar to the number and rate in 2008 (1.9 million or 0.7 percent) but were lower than the estimates in 2006 (2.4 million or 1.0 percent).

- Hallucinogens were used in the past month by 1.3 million persons (0.5 percent) aged 12 or older in 2009, including 760,000 (0.3 percent) who had used Ecstasy. The number and percentage of Ecstasy users increased between 2008 (555,000 or 0.2 percent) and 2009.

- In 2009, there were 7.0 million (2.8 percent) persons aged 12 or older who used prescription- type psychotherapeutic drugs nonmedically in the past month. These estimates were higher than in 2008 (6.2 million or 2.5 percent), but similar to estimates in 2007 (6.9 million or 2.8 percent).

- The number of past month methamphetamine users decreased between 2006 and 2008, but then increased in 2009. The numbers were 731,000 (0.3 percent) in 2006, 529,000 (0.2 percent) in

2007, 314,000 (0.1 percent) in 2008, and 502,000 (0.2 percent) in 2009.

- Among youths aged 12 to 17, the current illicit drug use rate increased from 2008 (9.3 percent) to 2009 (10.0 percent). Between 2002 and 2008, the rate declined from 11.6 to 9.3 percent.

- The rate of current marijuana use among youths aged 12 to 17 decreased from 8.2 percent in 2002 to 6.7 percent in 2006, remained unchanged at 6.7 percent in 2007 and 2008, then increased to 7.3 percent in 2009.

- Among youths aged 12 to 17, the rate of nonmedical use of prescription-type drugs declined from 4.0 percent in 2002 to

- 2.9 percent in 2008, then held steady at 3.1 percent in 2009.

- The rate of current Ecstasy use among youths aged 12 to 17 declined from 0.5 percent in 2002 to 0.3 percent in 2004, remained at that level through 2007, then increased to 0.5 percent in 2009.

- Between 2008 and 2009, the rate of current use of illicit drugs among young adults aged 18 to 25 increased from 19.6 to 21.2 percent, driven largely by an increase in marijuana use (from 16.5 to 18.1 percent).

- From 2002 to 2009, there was an increase among young adults aged 18 to 25 in the rate of current nonmedical use of prescription-type drugs (from 5.5 to 6.3 percent), driven primarily by an increase in pain reliever misuse (from 4.1 to 4.8 percent). There were decreases in the use of cocaine (from 2.0 to 1.4 percent) and methamphetamine (from 0.6 to 0.2 percent).

- Among those aged 50 to 59, the rate of past month illicit drug use increased from 2.7 percent in 2002 to 6.2 percent in 2009. This trend partially reflects the aging into this age group of the baby boom cohort, whose lifetime rate of illicit drug use is higher than those of older cohorts.

- Among persons aged 12 or older in 2008-2009 who used pain relievers nonmedically in the past 12 months, 55.3 percent got the drug they most recently used from a friend or relative for free. Another 17.6 percent reported they got the drug from one doctor. Only 4.8 percent got pain relievers from a drug dealer or other stranger, and 0.4 percent bought them on the Internet. Among those who reported getting the pain reliever from a friend or relative for free, 80.0 percent reported in a follow-up question that the friend or relative had obtained the drugs from just one doctor.

- Among unemployed adults aged 18 or older in 2009, 17.0 percent were current illicit drug users, which was higher than the 8.0 percent of those employed full time and 11.5 percent of those employed part time. However, most illicit drug users were employed. Of the 19.3 million current illicit drug users aged 18 or older in 2009, 12.9 million (66.6 percent) were employed either full or part time. The number of unemployed illicit drug users increased from 1.3 million in 2007 to 1.8 million in 2008 and 2.5 million in 2009, primarily because of an overall increase in the number of unemployed persons.

- In 2009, 10.5 million persons aged 12 or older reported driving under the influence of illicit drugs during the past year. This corresponds to 4.2 percent of the population aged 12 or older, which is similar to the rate in 2008 (4.0 percent) and the rate in 2002 (4.7 percent). In 2009, the rate was highest among young adults aged 18 to 25 (12.8 percent).

Alcohol Use

Slightly more than half of Americans aged 12 or older reported being current drinkers of alcohol in the 2009 survey (51.9 percent). This translates to an estimated 130.6 million people, which is similar to the 2008 estimate of 129.0 million people (51.6 percent).

In 2009, nearly one quarter (23.7 percent) of persons aged 12 or older participated in binge drinking. This translates to about 59.6 million people. The rate in 2009 is similar to the estimate in 2008. Binge drinking is defined as having five or more drinks on the same occasion on at least 1 day in the 30 days prior to the survey.

In 2009, heavy drinking was reported by 6.8 percent of the population aged 12 or older, or 17.1 million people. This rate was similar to the rate of heavy drinking in 2008. Heavy drinking is defined as binge drinking on at least 5 days in the past 30 days.

Among young adults aged 18 to 25 in 2009, the rate of binge drinking was 41.7 percent, and the rate of heavy drinking was 13.7 percent. These rates were similar to the rates in 2008.

The rate of current alcohol use among youths aged 12 to 17 was 14.7 percent in 2009, which is similar to the 2008 rate (14.6 percent). Youth binge and heavy drinking rates in 2009 (8.8 and 2.1 percent) were also similar to rates in 2008 (8.8 and 2.0 percent).

Past month and binge drinking rates among underage persons (aged 12 to 20) declined between 2002 and 2008, but then remained unchanged between 2008 (26.4 and 17.4 percent) and 2009 (27.2 and 18.1 percent).

Among persons aged 12 to 20, past month alcohol use rates in 2009 were 16.1 percent among Asians, 20.4 percent among blacks, 22.0 percent among American Indians or Alaska Natives, 25.1 percent among Hispanics, 27.5 percent among those reporting two or more races, and 30.4 percent among whites.

In 2009, 55.9 percent of current drinkers aged 12 to 20 reported that their last use of alcohol in the past month occurred in someone else's home, and 29.2 percent reported that it had occurred in their own home. About one third (30.3 percent) paid for the alcohol the last time they drank, including 9.0 percent who purchased the alcohol themselves and 21.3 percent who gave money to someone else to purchase it. Among those who did not pay for the alcohol they last drank, 37.1 percent got it from an unrelated person aged 21 or older, 19.9 percent from another person younger than 21 years old, and 20.6 percent from a parent, guardian, or other adult family member.

In 2009, an estimated 12.0 percent of persons aged 12 or older drove under the influence of alcohol at least once in the past year. This percentage has dropped since 2002, when it was 14.2 percent. The rate of driving under the influence of alcohol was highest among persons aged 21 to 25 (24.8 percent).

Tobacco Use

In 2009, an estimated 69.7 million Americans aged 12 or older were current (past month) users of a tobacco product. This represents 27.7 percent of the population in that age range. In addition, 58.7 million persons (23.3 percent of the population) were current cigarette smokers; 13.3 million (5.3 percent) smoked cigars; 8.6 million (3.4 percent) used smokeless tobacco; and 2.1 million (0.8 percent) smoked tobacco in pipes.

Between 2002 and 2009, past month use of any tobacco product decreased from 30.4 to 27.7 percent, and past month cigarette use declined from 26.0 to 23.3 percent. Rates of past month use of cigars, smokeless tobacco, and pipe tobacco in 2009 were similar to corresponding rates in 2002.

The rate of past month tobacco use among 12 to 17 year olds remained steady from 2008 to 2009 (11.4 and 11.6 percent, respectively). The rate of past month cigarette use among 12 to 17 year olds also remained steady between 2008 and 2009 (9.1 and 8.9 percent, respectively) but declined since 2002 when the rate was 13.0 percent. However, past month smokeless tobacco use among youths increased from 2.0 percent in 2002 to 2.3 percent in 2009.

Initiation of Substance Use (Incidence, or First-Time Use) within the Past 12 Months

In 2009, an estimated 3.1 million persons aged 12 or older used an illicit drug for the first time within the past 12 months. This averages to about 8,500 initiates per day and is similar to the estimate for 2008 (2.9 million). A majority of these past year illicit drug initiates reported that their first drug was marijuana (59.1 percent). Nearly one third initiated with psychotherapeutics (28.6 percent, including 17.1 percent with pain relievers, 8.6 percent with tranquilizers, 2.0 percent with stimulants, and 1.0 percent with sedatives). A sizable proportion reported inhalants (9.8 percent) as their first illicit drug, and a small proportion used hallucinogens as their first drug (2.1 percent).

In 2009, the illicit drug categories with the largest number of past year initiates among persons aged 12 or older were marijuana use (2.4 million) and nonmedical use of pain relievers (2.2 million). These estimates were not significantly different from the numbers in 2008.

However, the number of marijuana initiates increased between 2007 (2.1 million) and 2009 (2.4 million).

In 2009, the average age of marijuana initiates among persons aged 12 to 49 was 17.0 years, significantly lower than the average age of marijuana initiates in 2008 (17.8 years), but similar to that in 2002 (17.0 years).

The number of past year initiates of methamphetamine among persons aged 12 or older was 154,000 in 2009. This estimate was significantly higher than the estimate in 2008 (95,000), but lower than the estimate in 2002 (299,000).

There was a significant increase in the number of past year initiates of Ecstasy between 2008 and 2009, from 894,000 to 1.1 million. The estimate was 1.2 million in 2002, declined to 642,000 in 2003, and nearly doubled between 2005 (615,000) and 2009.

The number of past year cocaine initiates declined from 1.0 million in 2002 to 617,000 in 2009. The number of initiates of crack cocaine declined during this period from 337,000 to 94,000.

In 2009, there were 180,000 persons who used heroin for the first time within the past year, significantly more than the average annual number from 2002 to 2008. Estimates during those years ranged from 91,000 to 118,000 per year.

Most (85.5 percent) of the 4.6 million past year alcohol initiates were younger than 21 at the time of initiation.

The number of persons aged 12 or older who smoked cigarettes for the first time within the past 12 months was 2.5 million in 2009, similar to the estimate in 2008 (2.4 million), but significantly higher than the estimate for 2002 (1.9 million). Most new smokers in 2009 were younger than 18 when they first smoked cigarettes (58.8 percent or 1.5 million).

The number of persons aged 12 and older who used smokeless tobacco for the first time within the past year increased from 951,000 in 2002 to 1.5 million in 2009.

Youth Prevention-Related Measures

Perceived risk is measured by NSDUH as the percentage reporting that there is great risk in the substance use behavior. The percentage of youths aged 12 to 17 perceiving great risk in smoking marijuana once or twice a week increased from 51.5 percent in 2002 to 55.0 percent in

2005, but dropped to 49.3 percent in 2009. Between 2002 and 2008, the percentages who reported great risk in smoking one or more packs of cigarettes per day increased from 63.1 to 69.7 percent, but in 2009 the percentage dropped to 65.8 percent.

Almost half (49.9 percent) of youths aged 12 to 17 reported in 2009 that it would be "fairly easy" or "very easy" for them to obtain marijuana if they wanted some. Approximately one in five reported it would be easy to get cocaine (20.9 percent). About one in seven (13.5 percent) indicated that LSD would be "fairly" or "very" easily available, and 12.9 percent reported easy availability for heroin. Between 2002 and 2009, there were declines in the perceived availability for all four drugs.

A majority of youths aged 12 to 17 (90.5 percent) in 2009 reported that their parents would strongly disapprove of their trying marijuana or hashish once or twice. Current marijuana use was much less prevalent among youths who perceived strong parental disapproval for trying marijuana or hashish once or twice than for those who did not (4.8 vs. 31.3 percent).

In 2009, almost four fifths (77.0 percent) reported having seen or heard drug or alcohol prevention messages from sources outside of school, lower than in 2002 (83.2 percent). The percentage of school-enrolled youths reporting that they had seen or heard prevention messages at school also declined during this period, from 78.8 to 74.9 percent.

Substance Dependence, Abuse, and Treatment

In 2009, an estimated 22.5 million persons (8.9 percent of the population aged 12 or older) were classified with substance dependence or abuse in the past year based on criteria specified in the *Diagnostic and Statistical Manual of Mental Disorders*, 4th edition (DSM- IV). Of these, 3.2 million were classified with dependence on or abuse of both alcohol and illicit drugs, 3.9 million were dependent on or abused illicit drugs but not alcohol, and 15.4 million were dependent on or abused alcohol but not illicit drugs.

Between 2002 and 2009, the number of persons with substance dependence or abuse was stable (22.0 million in 2002 and 22.5 million in 2009).

The specific illicit drugs that had the highest levels of past year dependence or abuse in 2009 were marijuana (4.3 million), pain relievers

(1.9 million), and cocaine (1.1 million). The number of persons with marijuana dependence or abuse has not changed since 2002, but the number with pain reliever dependence or abuse has increased (from 1.5 million to 1.9 million) and the number with cocaine dependence or abuse has declined (from 1.5 million to 1.1 million).

In 2009, adults aged 21 or older who had first used alcohol at age 14 or younger were more than 6 times as likely to be classified with alcohol dependence or abuse than adults who had their first drink at age 21 or older (16.5 vs. 2.5 percent).

The rate of substance dependence or abuse for males aged 12 or older in 2009 was nearly twice as high as the rate for females (11.9 vs. 6.1 percent). Among youths aged 12 to 17, however, the rate of substance dependence or abuse among males (6.7 percent) was similar to the rate among females (7.4 percent).

Between 2002 and 2009, the percentage of youths aged 12 to 17 with substance dependence or abuse declined from 8.9 to 7.0 percent.

Treatment need is defined as having a substance use disorder or receiving treatment at a specialty facility (hospital inpatient, drug or alcohol rehabilitation, or mental health centers) within the past 12 months. In 2009, 23.5 million persons aged 12 or older needed treatment for an illicit drug or alcohol use problem (9.3 percent of persons aged 12 or older). Of these, 2.6 million (1.0 percent of persons aged 12 or older and 11.2 percent of those who needed treatment) received treatment at a specialty facility. Thus, 20.9 million persons
(8.3 percent of the population aged 12 or older) needed treatment for an illicit drug or alcohol use problem but did not receive treatment at a specialty substance abuse facility in the past year.

Of the 20.9 million persons aged 12 or older in 2009 who were classified as needing substance use treatment but did not receive treatment at a specialty facility in the past year, 1.1 million persons
(5.1 percent) reported that they felt they needed treatment for their illicit drug or alcohol use problem. Of these 1.1 million persons who felt they needed treatment, 371,000 (34.9 percent) reported that they made an effort to get treatment, and 693,000 (65.1 percent) reported making no effort to get treatment.

Selected and Annotated Sources:

SECTION I

- Medication prescribed by a doctor—does not include over the counter medication.

- http://usgovinfo.about.com/od/healthcare/a/usmedicated.htm

- Almost Half of Americans Take At Least One Prescription Drug, Half of Elderly Take Three or More by Robert Longley, About.com Guide 1/31/2011

- The book will be available in print or as an e-book for electronic readers or computers

- The Substance Abuse and Mental Health Services Administration's (SAMHSA's) National Survey on Drug Use and Health in 2006.

CHAPTER ONE:

- U.S. Department of Health and Human Services: Substance Abuse And Mental Health Services Administration Center For Substance Abuse: Prevention: Substance Abuse Prevention Dollars And Cents: A Cost-Benefit Analysis http://store. samhsa.gov/shin/content/SMA07-4298/ SMA07-4298.pdf

- The Benefits and Costs of Drug Use Prevention, Rand Corporation

- http://www.rand.org/pubs/research_briefs/RB6007/index1. html.//

- http://w.teendrugabuse.us/teensmoking.html 10.

- Perhaps the best analogy for this effect is the "Here's your brain on drugs/fried eggs" public service announcement that is still running after 30 years.

CHAPTER TWO

- Author Note: The DSM may have new changes in the near future-this avoids dating the book.

- Blumenthal DM, Gold MS. (2010) Neurobiology of food addiction. Curr Opin Clin Nutr Metab Care, 13(4): 359-365.

CHAPTER THREE

- http://www.vitamist.com/Articles.asp?ID=137&?Click=3634

- Safe pain killers without some of aspirin's side effects have evolved and reduced the potential for addiction or organ damage if used properly. These include ibuprofen and acetaminophen.

- The latest health data collected by the Centers for Disease Control and Prevention's (CDC) National Center for Health Statistics and dozens of other Federal health agencies, academic and professional health associations, and international health organizations.

- Some discounted medical systems widely practiced in India like Ayurvedic treatments had been discounted by NIH until recently.

- Narcotic Drugs, by Dr. Anil Aggrawal, National Book Trust, May, 1995 New Delhi, India

- Vagnini, Frederic, MD, Chilnick, Lawrence D., Beating the Cardio- Diabetic Connection, FW Enterprise, New York, 2011.

- Narcon international

- http://www.narconon.org/drug-information/egypt-drug-addiction.html. http://www.localhistories.org/medicine. html 26. Ibid 5 27. A Brief History Of Medicine By Tim Lambert

- http://www.localhistories.org/medicine.html 28. Ibid 8

- http://www.ars-rhetorica.net/Queen/Volum...http://www.henriettesherbal.com/eclectic

- Patent medicines in their original sense referred to medications whose ingredients had been granted government protection for exclusivity. The Constitution (Article I, Section 8, Clause 8) granted Congress the power to regulate such protections; a Patent Office was established in 1790

- http://www.powerweb.net/bbock/war/amputate.html 32. http://www.ncbi.nlm.nih.gov/pubmed/18176164 33. www.u-s-history.com/pages/h917.html 34. (The Meat Inspection Act was passed in 1911.)

- Drug Use and Addiction in War: Tom Langdale, http://www.highestfive.com/combat/drug-use-and-addiction-in-war/ http://www.historylearningsite.co.uk/history_of_medicine. htm 39. Ibid 17

- http://www.nlm.nih.gov/hmd/ http://www. historylearningsite.co.uk/history_of_medicine.htm

CHAPTER FOUR

- A combination of substances the users thought were healing and a hot compress—unfortunately these were more deadly than helpful.

- The survey is the primary source of information on the use of illicit drugs, alcohol, and tobacco in the civilian, noninstitutionalized population of the United States aged 12 years old or older. The survey interviews approximately 67,500 persons each year. Unless otherwise noted, all comparisons in this report described using terms such as "increased," "decreased," or "more than" are statistically significant at the .05 level.

- Substance Abuse and Mental Health Services Administration. (2010). Results from the 2009 National Survey on Drug Use and Health: Volume I. Summary of National Findings (Office of Applied Studies, NSDUH Series H-38A, HHS Publication No. SMA 10-4586Findings). Rockville, MD.

- Thomas Jefferson and George Washington, certainly agriculture successes, both farmed marijuana

- Why Is Marijuana Illegal? www.DrugWarRant.com, Pete Guither

- http://www.naihc.org/hemp_information/hemp_facts.html

- Cermak, Timmen, The California Society of Addiction Medicine, Introduction to CSAM's Evidence-Based Information on Cannabis/Marijuana http://www.csamasam. org/newsletter. vp.html, Fall 2010

- Working at Hebrew University in Jerusalem. 49. Ibid 45 50. Ibid 45

- Gold et. al, Marijuana, Gabbards Treatments of Psychiatric Disorders, American Psychiatric Publishing, Inc. 4th Edition, pp. 247-255, Arlington, VA., 2007

- http://www.time.com/time/nation/ article/0,8599,1884956,00. html#ixzz1GluY6qAN

- http://www.time.com/time/nation/ article/0,8599,1884956,00. html#ixzz1GlvFv3vh

- March 13, 2009 54.

- Patricia O'Malley, PhD, RN, CNS, "Prescription and Over-the-Counter Drug and Substance Abuse: Something Available for Every Age, Anytime and Anywhere", Clinical Nurse Specialist, copyright 2010, Williams & Wilkins

- Pain is judged on a scale of 1-10, but is reported subjectively by the patient.

- National Ambulatory Medical Care Survey: 2008 Summary Tables, tables 22, 23, 24

- http://www.teenhelp.com/teen-drug-abuse/

- http://www.teendrugabuse.us/over_the_counter_drug_abuse. htm

- Over-the-Counter Drug Abuse 61. Ibid 59 62. Author interview 63. Ibid 59

CHAPTER FIVE

- http://www.aacap.org/cs/root/facts_for_families/children_ of_ alcoholics American Academy of Child and Adolescent Psychiatry

- United Nations Demographic Surveys

- www.cdc.gov/alcohol/fact-sheets/underage-drinking.htm July 2010

- www.teenhelp.com

- Using Teachable Moments To Talk With Teens About Sex, Posted in Birth Control, Family Planning, STD & HIV Safety

- Finding the Teachable Moments: Adapted from: "A Parent's Guide to Discussing Dating: Teenage Daughters". By Karen Ray ©2002 Pagewise. http://www.laughyourway.com/teens/ finding- the-teachable-moments/

SECTION II

- Author experience.

- http://www.teendrugabuse.us/over_the_counter_drug_abuse. htm

- Over-the-Counter Drug Abuse 73. Ibid 72 74. Ibid 32 75. Ibid 32

- These data are from the 2009 Monitoring the Future survey, funded by the National Institute on Drug Abuse, National Institutes of Health, Department of Health and Human Services, and conducted annually by the University of Michigan's Institute for Social Research. The survey has tracked 12th-graders' illicit drug use and related attitudes since 1975; in 1991, 8th- and 10th-graders were added to the study. The latest data are on line at www. drugabuse.gov.

- www.drugabuse.gov. National Institute on Drug Abuse, National Institutes of Health

- Data are from the 2009 Monitoring the Future survey, funded by the National Institute on Drug Abuse, National Institutes of Health, Department of Health and Human Services, and conducted annually by the University of Michigan's Institute for Social Research. The survey has tracked 12th-graders' illicit drug use and related attitudes since 1975; in 1991, 8th- and 10th-graders were added to the study.

- "Lifetime" refers to use at least once during a respondent's lifetime. "Past year" refers to use at least once during the year preceding an individual's response to the survey. "Past month" refers to use at least once during the 30 days preceding an individual's response to the survey.

- http://www.whitehousedrugpolicy.gov/publications/ international/ factsht/internl_heroin_mkt.html

- http://www.nida.nih.gov/infofacts/heroin.html

- http://www.heroin-effects.com/

- Monitoring The Future Study, University of Michigan, 2011

- www.drugabuse.com, National Institute on Drug Abuse. InfoFacts: Anabolic Steroids

- www.monitoringthefuture.org 2010 93. www.teendrugabuse. us/ teensmoking.html

- Chavkin, C., Sud, S., Jin, W. et al. Salvinorin A, an active component of the hallucinogenic sage Salvia divinorum is a highly efficacious kappa-opioid receptor agonist: structural and functional considerations. J Pharmacol Exp Ther. 308:1197– 203, 2004. 2 Harding, W.W.

Appendix B: Glossary from NIDA For Teens: The Science Behind Drug Abuse. National Institute on Drug Abuse, May, 2011

http://teens.drugabuse.gov/utilities/glossary.php

A

AIDS (Acquired Immunodeficiency Syndrome): A condition characterized by a defect in the body's natural immunity to diseases. Individuals who suffer from it are at risk for severe illnesses that are usually not a threat to anyone whose immune system is working properly.

Addiction: A chronic, relapsing disease characterized by compulsive drug-seeking and abuse and by long-lasting chemical changes in the brain.

Adrenal glands: Glands, located above each, kidney that secrete hormones, e.g., adrenaline.

Amphetamine: Stimulant drugs whose effects are very similar to cocaine.

Amyl nitrite: A yellowish oily volatile liquid used in certain diagnostic procedures and prescribed to some patients for heart pain. Illegally diverted ampules of amyl nitrite are called "poppers" or "snappers" on the street.

Anabolic effects: Drug-induced growth or thickening of the body's nonreproductive tract tissues-including skeletal muscle, bones, the larynx, and vocal cords-and decrease in body fat.

Analgesics: A group of medications that reduce pain.

Anesthetic: An agent that causes insensitivity to pain and is used for surgeries and other medical procedures.

Androgenic effects: A drug's effects upon the growth of the male reproductive tract and the development of male secondary sexual characteristics.

Aplastic anemia: A disorder that occurs when the bone marrow produces too few of all three types of blood cells: red blood cells, white blood cells, and platelets.

Axon terminal: The structure at the end of an axon that produces and releases chemicals (neurotransmitters) to transmit the neuron's message across the synapse.

Axon: The fiber-like extension of a neuron by which the cell carries information to target cells.

B

Benzene: A volatile liquid solvent found in gasoline.

Bind: The attaching of a neurotransmitter or other chemical to a receptor. The neurotransmitter is said to "bind" to the receptor. Brainstem: The major route by which the forebrain sends information to, and receives information from, the spinal cord and peripheral nerves. Butane: A substance found in lighter fluid. Butyl nitrite: An illegal substance that is often packaged and sold in small bottles; also referred to as "poppers"

C

Cannabinoid receptor: The receptor in the brain that recognizes anandamide and THC, the active ingredient in marijuana.

Cannabinoids: Chemicals that help control mental and physical processes when produced naturally by the body and that produce intoxication and other effects when absorbed from marijuana.

Cannabis: The botanical name for the plant from which marijuana comes.

Carcinogen: Any substance that causes cancer.

Cardiovascular system: The heart and blood vessels.

Cell body (or soma): The central structure of a neuron, which contains the cell nucleus. The cell body contains the molecular machinery that regulates the activity of the neuron.

Central nervous system: The brain and spinal cord.

Cerebellum: A portion of the brain that helps regulate posture, balance, and coordination.

Cerebral cortex: Region of the brain responsible for cognitive functions including reasoning, mood, and perception of stimuli.

Cerebral hemispheres: The two specialized halves of the brain. The left hemisphere is specialized for speech, writing, language, and calculation; the right hemisphere is specialized for spatial abilities, face recognition in vision, and some aspects of music perception and production.

Cerebrum: The upper part of the brain consisting of the left and right hemispheres.

Chloroform: A colorless volatile liquid used as a medical anesthetic gas.

Chronic: Refers to a disease or condition that persists over a long period of time.

Coca: The plant, Erythroxylon, from which cocaine is derived. Also refers to the leaves of this plant.

Cocaethylene: A substance created in the body when cocaine and alcohol are used together; chemically similar to cocaine. Cocaine: A highly addictive stimulant drug derived from the coca plant that produces profound feelings of pleasure.

Crack: "Slang" term for a smokeable form of cocaine.

Craving: A powerful, often uncontrollable desire for drugs.

Cyclohexyl nitrite: A chemical found in substances marketed as room deodorizers.

D

Dendrite: The specialized branches that extend from a neuron's cell body and function to receive messages from other neurons.

Depressants: Drugs that relieve anxiety and produce sleep. Depressants include barbiturates, benzodiazepines, and alcohol.

Dopamine: A brain chemical, classified as a neurotransmitter, found in regions of the brain that regulate movement, emotion, motivation, and pleasure.

Drug: A chemical compound or substance that can alter the structure and function of the body. Psychoactive drugs affect the function of the brain, and some of these may be illegal to use and possess.

Drug abuse: The use of illegal drugs or the inappropriate use of legal drugs. The repeated use of drugs to produce pleasure, to alleviate stress, or to alter or avoid reality (or all three).

E

Ecstasy (MDMA): A chemically modified amphetamine that has hallucinogenic as well as stimulant properties.

Emphysema: A lung disease in which tissue deterioration results in increased air retention and reduced exchange of gases. The result is difficult breathing and shortness of breath. It is often caused by smoking.

Endogenous: Something produced by the brain or body.

Ether: A volatile liquid with a characteristic odor. Used as a medical anesthetic gas.

Euphoria: A feeling of well-being or elation.

F

Fluorinated hydrocarbons: Gases or liquids commonly found in refrigerants, fire extinguishers, solvents, and anesthetics. Freon is one class of fluorinated hydrocarbons.

Forebrain: The largest division of the brain, which includes the cerebral cortex and basal ganglia. It is credited with the highest intellectual functions.

Frontal lobe: One of the four divisions of each cerebral hemisphere. The frontal lobe is important for controlling movement and associating the functions of other cortical areas.

H

Hallucinations: Perceptions of something (such as a visual image or a sound) that does not really exist. Hallucinations usually arise from a disorder of the nervous system or in response to drugs (such as LSD).

Hallucinogens: A diverse group of drugs that alter perceptions, thoughts, and feelings. Hallucinogenic drugs include LSD, mescaline, MDMA (ecstasy), PCP, and psilocybin (magic mushrooms).

Halothane: Medical anesthetic gas.

Hepatitis: Inflammation of the liver.

Heroin: The potent, widely abused opiate that produces addiction. It consists of two morphine molecules linked together chemically.

Hexane: A hydrocarbon volatile liquid found in glue or gasoline.

Hippocampus: An area of the brain crucial for learning and memory.

HIV (Human Immunodeficiency Virus): The virus that causes AIDS (Acquired Immunodeficiency Syndrome).

Hormone: A chemical substance formed in glands in the body and carried in the blood to organs and tissues, where it influences function, structure, and behavior.

Hypothalamus: The part of the brain that controls many bodily functions, including feeding, drinking, and the release of many hormones.

I

Ingestion: The act of taking in food or other material into the body through the mouth.

Inhalant: Any drug administered by breathing in its vapors. Inhalants commonly are organic solvents, such as glue and paint thinner or anesthetic gases, such as ether and nitrous oxide.

Inhalation: The act of administering a drug or combination of drugs by nasal or oral respiration. Also, the act of drawing air or other substances into the lungs. Nicotine in tobacco smoke enters the body by inhalation.

Injection: A method of administering a substance such as a drug into the skin, subcutaneous tissue, muscle, blood vessels, or body cavities, usually by means of a needle.

L

Limbic system: A set of brain structures that generates our feelings, emotions, and motivations. It is also important in learning and memory.

LSD (lysergic acid diethylamide): An hallucinogenic drug that acts on the serotonin receptor.

M

Marijuana: A drug, usually smoked but can be eaten, that is made from the flowers and leaves of the cannabis plant. The main psychoactive ingredient is THC.

Medication: A drug that is used to treat an illness or disease according to established medical guidelines.

Metabolism: The processes by which the body breaks things down or alters them so they can be eliminated.

Methamphetamine: A commonly abused, potent stimulant drug that is part of a larger family of amphetamines.

Methylphenidate (Ritalin®): Methylphenidate is a central nervous system stimulant. It has effects similar to, but more potent than, caffeine and less potent than amphetamines. It has a notably calming and "focusing" effect on those with ADHD, particularly children.

Musculoskeletal system: The muscles, bones, tendons, and ligaments.

Myelin: Fatty material that surrounds and insulates axons of most neurons.

N

Neuron (nerve cell): A unique type of cell found in the brain and body, specialized to process and transmit information.

Neurotransmission: The process that occurs when a neuron releases neurotransmitters to communicate with another neuron across the synapse.

Neurotransmitter: A chemical produced by neurons to carry messages to other neurons.

Nicotine: The addictive drug in tobacco. Nicotine activates a specific type of acetylcholine receptor.

Nitrites: A special class of inhalants that act primarily to dilate blood vessels and relax the muscles. Whereas other inhalants are used to alter mood, nitrites are used primarily as sexual enhancers. (See also amyl nitrite and butyl nitrite).

Nitrous oxide: Medical anesthetic gas, especially used in dentistry. Also called "laughing gas". Found in whipped cream dispensers and gas cylinders.

Noradrenaline: A chemical neurotransmitter that is made in the brain and can affect the heart.

Nucleus: A cluster or group of nerve cells that is dedicated to performing its own special function(s). Nuclei are found in all parts of the brain but are called cortical fields in the cerebral cortex.

Nucleus accumbens: A part of the brain reward system, located in the limbic system, that processes information related to motivation and reward. Virtually all drugs of abuse act on the nucleus accumbens to reinforce drug taking.

O

Occipital lobe: The lobe of the cerebral cortex at the back of the head that includes the visual cortex.

P

Parietal lobe: One of the four subdivisions of the cerebral cortex; it is involved in sensory processes, attention, and language.

Physical dependence: An adaptive physiological state that occurs with regular drug use and results in a withdrawal syndrome when drug use is stopped; usually occurs with tolerance.

Polyneuropathy: Permanent change or malfunction of nerves. Sudden sniffing death; a type of death that can occur when inhaled fumes fill up the cells in the lungs with poisonous chemicals, leaving no room for the oxygen needed to breathe. This lack of oxygen can lead to suffocation, respiratory failure, and death.

Polyneuropathy: A drug that distorts perception, thought, and feeling. This term is typically used to refer to drugs with actions like those of LSD.

Psychoactive: Having a specific effect on the mind.

Psychoactive drug: A drug that changes the way the brain works.

R

Receptor: A large molecule that recognizes specific chemicals (normally neurotransmitters, hormones, and similar endogenous substances) and transmits the message carried by the chemical into the cell on which the receptor resides.

Relapse: In drug abuse, relapse is the resumption of drug use after trying to stop taking drugs. Relapse is a common occurrence in many chronic disorders, including addiction, that requires behavioral adjustments to treat effectively.

Reuptake: The process by which neurotransmitters are removed from the synapse by being "pumped" through transporters back into the axon terminals that first released them.

Reuptake pump (transporter): The large molecule that actually transports neurotransmitter molecules back into the axon terminals that released them.

Reward: The process that reinforces behavior. It is mediated at least in part by the release of dopamine into the nucleus accumbens. Human subjects report that reward is associated with feelings of pleasure.

Reward system (or brain reward system): A brain circuit that, when activated, reinforces behaviors. The circuit includes the dopamine-containing neurons of the ventral tegmental area, the nucleus accumbens, and part of the prefrontal cortex. The activation of this circuit causes feelings of pleasure.

Route of administration: The way a drug is put into the body. Drugs can enter the body by eating, drinking, inhaling, injecting, snorting, smoking, or absorbing a drug through mucous membranes.

Rush: A surge of pleasure that rapidly follows administration of some drugs.

S

Serotonin: A neurotransmitter that regulates many functions, including mood, appetite, and sensory perception.

Sex hormones: Hormones that are found in higher quantities in one sex than in the other. Male sex hormones are the androgens, which include testosterone; and the female sex hormones are the estrogens and progesterone.

Stimulants: A class of drugs that elevates mood, increases feelings of well-being, and increases energy and alertness. These drugs produce euphoria and are powerfully rewarding. Stimulants include cocaine, Methamphetamine, and methylphenidate (Ritalin).

Synapse: The site where presynaptic and postsynaptic neurons communicate with each other.

Synaptic space (or synaptic cleft): The intercellular space between the presynaptic and postsynaptic neurons.

T

Temporal lobe: The lobe of the cerebral cortex at the side of the head that hears and interprets music and language.

Tetrahydrocannabinol: See THC.

Thalamus: Located deep within the brain, the thalamus is the key relay station for sensory information flowing into the brain, filtering out important messages from the mass of signals entering the brain.

THC: Delta-9-tetrahydrocannabinol; the main active ingredient in marijuana, which acts on the brain to produce its effects.

Tobacco: A plant widely cultivated for its leaves, which are used primarily for smoking; the tabacum species is the major source of tobacco products.

Tolerance: A condition in which higher doses of a drug are required to produce the same effect as during initial use; often leads to physical dependence.

Toluene: A light colorless liquid solvent found in many commonly abused inhalants, including airplane glue, paint sprays, and paint and nail polish removers.

Transporter: A light colorless liquid solvent found in many commonly abused inhalants, including airplane glue, paint sprays, and paint and nail polish removers.

Trichloroethylene: A liquid used as a solvent and in medicine as an anesthetic and analgesic. Found in cleaning fluid and correction fluid.

V

Ventral tegmental area (VTA): The group of dopamine-containing neurons that make up a key part of the brain reward system. These neurons extend axons to the nucleus accumbens and the prefrontal cortex.

Vertigo: The sensation of dizziness.
Vesicle: A membranous sac within an axon terminal that stores and releases neurotransmitter.

W

Withdrawal: Symptoms that occur after chronic use of a drug is reduced or stopped.

References:

National Institute on Drug Abuse. NIDA Research Report-Marijuana Abuse, Glossary http://www.drugabuse.gov/ResearchReports/Marijuana/Marijuana6. html#glossary: NIH Pub. No. 02-3859. Bethesda, MD: NIDA, NIH, DHHS. October 2002.

National Institute on Drug Abuse. NIDA Research Report-Steroid Abuse and Addiction, Glossary http://www.drugabuse.gov/ResearchReports/Steroids/ anabolicsteroids5. html#glossary: NIH Pub. No. 00-3721. Bethesda, MD: NIDA, NIH, DHHS. Printed 1991. Reprinted 1994, 1996. Revised April 2000.

National Institute on Drug Abuse. NIDA Research Report-Nicotine Addiction, Glossary http://www.drugabuse.gov/researchreports/nicotine/nicotine5. html#glossary: NIH Pub. No. 01-4342. Bethesda, MD: NIDA, NIH, DHHS. Printed July, 1998. Reprinted August 2001.

National Institute on Drug Abuse. NIDA Research Report-Hallucinogens and Dissociative Drugs, Glossary http://www.drugabuse.gov/ResearchReports/ hallucinogens/halluc5.html: NIH Pub. No. 01-4209. Bethesda, MD: NIDA, NIH, DHHS. Printed March 2001.

National Institute on Drug Abuse. The Brain: Understanding Neurobiology Through the Study of Addiction, Glossary http://www.drugabuse.gov/ Curriculum/HSCurriculum.html: NIH Pub. No. 00-4871. Bethesda, MD: NIDA, NIH, DHHS. Printed 2000.

National Institute on Drug Abuse. NIDA Research Report- Cocaine Abuse and Addiction, Glossary http://www.drugabuse.gov/ResearchReports/Cocaine/ cocaine5.html#glossary: NIH Pub. No. 99-4342, Bethesda, MD: NIDA, NIH, DHHS. Printed May 1999. Revised November 2004

National Institute on Drug Abuse. NIDA InfoFacts- Methylphenidate (Ritalin) http://www.drugabuse.gov/Infofacts/ritalin.html:
National Institute on Drug Abuse. NIDA InfoFacts: Drug Abuse and AIDS http://www.drugabuse.gov/Infofacts/drugabuse.html:

National Institute on Drug Abuse. NIDA Research Report- Inhalants Abuse http://www.drugabuse.gov/ResearchReports/Inhalants/: NIH Pub. No. 00-3818, Bethesda, MD: NIDA, NIH, DHHS. Printed 1994, Reprinted 1996, 1999. Revised July, 2000, Revised 2005

INDEX